100 Questions and Answers About Plastic Surgery

Diane Gerber, MD, FACS

Marie Czenko Kuechel, MA

JONES AND BARTLETT PUBLISHERS
Sudbury, Massachusetts
BOSTON   TORONTO   LONDON   SINGAPORE

World Headquarters

Jones and Bartlett
Publishers
40 Tall Pine Drive
Sudbury, MA 01776
info@jbpub.com
www.jbpub.com

Jones and Bartlett
Publishers Canada
2406 Nikanna Road
Mississauga, ON L5C 2W6
CANADA

Jones and Bartlett
Publishers International
Barb House, Barb Mews
London W6 7PA
UK

The authors, editor, and publisher have made every effort to provide accurate information. However, they are not responsible for errors, omissions, or for any outcomes related to the use of the contents of this book and take no responsibility for the use of the products described. Treatments and side effects described in this book may not be applicable to all patients; likewise, some patients may require a dose or experience a side effect that is not described herein. The reader should confer with his or her own physician regarding specific treatments and side effects. Drugs and medical devices are discussed that may have limited availability controlled by the Food and Drug Administration (FDA) for use only in a research study or clinical trial. The drug information presented has been derived from reference sources, recently published data, and pharmaceutical research data. Research, clinical practice, and government regulations often change the accepted standard in this field. When consideration is being given to use of any drug in the clinical setting, the health care provider or reader is responsible for determining FDA status of the drug, reading the package insert, reviewing prescribing information for the most up-to-date recommendations on dose, precautions, and contraindications, and determining the appropriate usage for the product. This is especially important in the case of drugs that are new or seldom used.

Library of Congress Cataloging-in-Publication Data

Gerber, Diane.
  100 questions and answers about plastic surgery / by Diane Gerber and Marie Czenko Kuechel.— 1st ed.
    p. cm.
  ISBN 0-7637-2632-X
  1. Surgery, Plastic—Miscellanea. 2. Surgery, Plastic—Popular works. I. Title: One hundred questions and answers about plastic surgery. II. Kuechel, Marie Czenko. III. Title.
  RD119.G47 2005
  617.9'52—dc22

                                                                          2004012085

Production Credits
Executive Editor: Jack Bruggeman
Production Manager: Amy Rose
Associate Production Editor: Renée Sekerak
Editorial Assistant: Kylah McNeill
Marketing Manager: Ed McKenna
Manufacturing Buyer: Therese Bräuer
Composition: Northeast Compositors
Cover Design: Kristin E. Ohlin
Printing and Binding: Malloy, Inc.
Cover Printing: Malloy, Inc.

Printed in the United States of America
08 07 06 05 04   10 9 8 7 6 5 4 3 2 1

Contents

Part 1: Plastic Surgery: Definitions and Desire   1

Questions 1-8 define what plastic surgery is and who are plastic surgery candidates, including:
- What is plastic surgery?
- Why should I consider having plastic surgery?
- Why wouldn't I consider having plastic surgery?
- What are realistic expectations?

Part 2: Plastic Surgery Providers   13

Questions 9-13 discuss the different types of appropriately credentialed plastic surgery providers, including:
- What defines a qualified plastic surgeon?
- What other credentials and factors should be considered?
- How can a qualified provider be found?

Part 3: Where to Begin   23

Questions 14-20 discuss selecting a provider to perform your plastic surgery and the process of consultation, including:
- How do I choose a physician to perform my surgery?
- What is involved in a consultation?
- What is informed consent?

Part 4: Paying for Plastic Surgery   35

Questions 21-26 define cost considerations for plastic surgery, including:
- Will insurance cover plastic surgery costs?
- Are there hidden costs?
- Can money be saved on a procedure?

Interest in cosmetic plastic surgery is at an all-time high. On television and radio, in magazines, and on the Internet there are programs, stories, and information about cosmetic plastic surgery. Much of this information is helpful. Unfortunately, some of it is not. Independent studies on patient interest indicate that the number of people considering cosmetic plastic surgery is very high. Because of this high level of interest, and the amount of sometimes confusing information, the need to have better informed cosmetic plastic surgery patients has never been greater. Fortunately, Diane Gerber, MD and Marie Czenko Kuechel have written *100 Questions and Answers About Plastic Surgery*.

This important book has been written jointly by a cosmetic plastic surgery advisor and journalist, an individual with many years of experience working with plastic surgeons, and an active practicing plastic surgeon, performing cosmetic plastic surgery for years in a highly competitive market. Marie Czenko Kuechel, MA and Dr. Diane Gerber have combined talents and skills to provide any patient interested in cosmetic surgery with an eminently readable book. The "100 Question and Answer" format walks prospective and active patients through the most commonly asked questions. The authors provide answers with appropriate references to validate the information. This is what is so often lacking in the Internet sources. The questions are formatted in clearly worded inquiries, obviously extracted from those answered through years of experience by Dr. Gerber. The answers are from her years of experience and influenced and formatted by Ms. Kuechel's writing as a consultant and journalist. This strong team has produced a text that will benefit all categories of patients interested in cosmetic plastic surgery. The side benefit will be to the practicing plastic surgeon, whose prospective patients will be better informed and prepared to make decisions, which will be lifelong. All will benefit from reading and understanding the 100 questions and answers provided in this welcome addition to the many self-help volumes available to prospective plastic surgery patients.

James H. Wells, MD, FACS
President
American Society of Plastic Surgeons®
2002-2003

When Marie Kuechel approached me to co-author this book, I knew it was a terrific opportunity to help people make more informed choices about plastic surgery. There is so much hype on TV and in magazines and newspapers, that it's easy for consumers to get carried away—to jump on the "bandwagon" without really considering their options. New techniques and procedures are touted all the time. Are they safe? Is there a better way to accomplish the same goal? What are the side effects? These factors must be considered. Safety, outcome, cost, medical history, family situation and lifestyle goals must be discussed and a surgeon must be chosen.

After completing college at Vassar and medical school at Columbia University College of Physicians and Surgeons, I pursued a residency in General Surgery at Northwestern University, knowing that plastic surgery was my ultimate goal. After three years of residency in General Surgery, I continued at Northwestern to complete an additional three-year residency in Plastic and Reconstructive Surgery. This, I might add, is not the case for every physician who practices cosmetic surgery. It is important for consumers to know that, only through the extensive surgical training received during similar dual surgical residencies, can a physician be board certified by the American Board of Plastic Surgery, the *only* board recognized by the American Board of Medical Specialties to certify surgeons in plastic, cosmetic, and reconstructive surgery.

In order for patients to get the best outcome, a surgeon needs an artistic sense in addition to technical skill. I explain to each patient that we need to set realistic goals and determine what procedures will create facial harmony. A keen eye, good judgment, the ability to listen and communicate, and surgical skills are necessary ingredients to get the desired outcome. This also holds true for determining aesthetic procedures relating to the breast and body.

Plastic surgery is a "feel good" profession. I strive to make people look better, more refreshed, a little younger. When they think that they look great, they often feel so much better about themselves. It's the best of all worlds, and I love coming into my office and surgical center every day.

As a media spokesperson for the American Society of Plastic Surgeons (ASPS) and the American Society for Aesthetic Plastic Surgery (ASAPS), I have the opportunity to continue my interest in public education. I firmly believe that the more knowledge a prospective patient has, the more satisfied that patient will be with the results of the procedure. If a patient comes into my office for a consultation and says, "Just make me look good," I see red flags. Consequently, we talk everything through very carefully and make sure we end up with realistic goals and expectations. Although aesthetic surgery can be a life-changing experience, in many cases, it doesn't change who you are inside.

Every person should have a copy of this book before considering aesthetic surgery. Ask the questions. If you don't get the answers, head for the door. It's your money, your body, and your emotions. Never settle for anything less than the best. You deserve it.

Diane L. Gerber, MD, FACS

Personal and Professional, Questions and Answers

I once thought I would make my career in sports broadcasting. Instead I have found myself specializing in a very different type of communication—medical communications and patient education. As much as my professional career path brought me somewhere I never expected, few of us set out in life knowing that one day we might consider plastic surgery. But my career has been immensely rewarding and I wouldn't trade it for the world, just like the fulfillment many people feel after undergoing plastic surgery.

My career didn't happen by chance—it required an education of my own, a dedication and compassion for both the needs of patients and physicians, and business, legal, and medical knowledge—plus a little introspection. So too, the decision for plastic surgery should not happen by chance unless it is in the treatment of trauma, disease, or birth defect. And even then, your circumstance, not your outcome, when plastic surgery is approached with education, sincerity, and candor.

I began my career in patient education and plastic surgery at the American Society for Plastic Surgeons®, the world's largest and leading organization devoted to the medical specialty of plastic surgery and to the professional excellence of board-certified plastic surgeons in the United States and Canada. Developing patient education for such a group at 24 years of age was a challenge I embraced. It set the foundation for what continues to be my passion—translating medical language into something that people can understand, embrace, and accept as reality. Information that helps physicians better communicate and patients more readily understand.

Throughout my career and association with the field of plastic surgery, countless people have asked what I have had "done". Early in my career, this is where introspect was required. Did I want to spend my professional life attached to what so many think of as the ultimate in vanity?

Decisions and Choices

I know I made the right decision. Each day I spend with qualified, caring, and compassionate providers of plastic surgery, and with the patients who are personally fulfilled through this amazing specialty of medicine, it is most obvious that there is no vanity here. This is the ultimate in confident people, personal fulfillment, and where science and artistry translate through medicine to enhance natural human beauty. The fulfillment of others is what fuels my dedication to elevating the role of plastic surgery with patients and the public. And these days, maintaining, much less elevating, the perception of plastic surgery in our society is truly a challenge.

Today, sensationalized media can easily misinform or misguide consumers. Unqualified providers often use slick advertising to appeal to insecurities. And, there are so many myths and fallacies about plastic surgery, and so many labels and illusions. Patients and those they love, as well as the public are often confused about the desire for plastic surgery, the providers of plastic surgery, the choices, the risks, and the rewards.

After spending more than a decade working in public and patient education in this incredible specialty of medicine, I can tell you the rewards of plastic surgery are real. No myth, no accident. From the reconstructive procedures that miraculously restore what nature or accident has denied, to the aesthetic procedures that enhance appearance and personal confidence—the rewards are real. But treatment is also real.

Just as any medical treatment has potential for complications and carries risk, so does plastic surgery. Minimizing risk and maximizing your rewards requires an educated, candid, and compliant patient, and a carefully selected, appropriately skilled provider.

Choices and Questions

Whether you are curious about or have the desire for plastic surgery, you should read this book before making the decision to consult with a qualified provider. I don't expect in 100 questions that every question can be answered. I can only expect to generate many more questions. Those additional questions can be answered through education and communication specific to you, and specifically from a qualified provider of plastic surgery. How do I know?

I speak not only from professional, but also from personal, experience. As much as I have worked in plastic surgery, I have been a patient. And for all of those who question what I have had "done"—that is my business alone, and that of my surgeon and co-author, Diane L. Gerber, MD, FACS.

The more important question you can ask me is why I have written this book: I believe in this industry, this specialty of medicine, and what it offers the human body *and* the human spirit.

I spent years talking and writing about the fulfillment that plastic surgery can provide individuals. That belief was fully validated when I made the choice to become a patient. Every day I am completely fulfilled by my choice for that one procedure that I know was absolutely right for me.

You can be fulfilled, too, if you are educated, realistic about the process, risks, and outcomes, and sincere in your desire. Plastic surgery is something you choose for no one but yourself. Media should not create or influence desire; authoritative, unbiased media should educate you. Your physician should not create or influence your desire; he or she should fully, candidly, and compassionately inform you about the appropriate treatment, your alternatives, and realistic outcomes, including risk. Those who love you should not make or influence your decision; they should support you, your desire, and any decision you make.

There is one message that I hope you keep with you, when reading this book and for life. *You* can be fulfilled in *your desire*. Whether is it is your decision to have plastic surgery or any decision you have to make in life, it is you who is in control. You must ask the questions. You must question the answers. And only you can make your own decisions.

For all of those whose motivation and intention is sincere, who believe in themselves and in those they love—may you always be fulfilled.

Marie Czenko Kuechel, MA

As I look back over the years from the time I was a fledgling medical student, I am gratified by the wonderful, intelligent, and caring people and organizations that have impacted my life and continue to support, encourage, and educate me. I've learned that it takes more than technical ability to excel in my profession. It takes the ability to learn from others, to communicate, and to empathize. Giving back to family, friends, patients, educators, colleagues, and people that I encounter on a daily basis helps me to put everything into perspective. I am grateful each and every day.

To my husband, Howard, and my son, Jim, thank you for your support and patience as I labored over this book. You know my love for you never falters.

My thanks to my parents who showed me the way, taught me to always strive for excellence, and who sacrificed to put me through so many years of schooling. I am eternally grateful.

A hearty thank you to my office staff, especially Arlene and Diane, who over the past 18 years have stood patiently by my side, always enthusiastic and supportive. You have helped me to build my practice into what it is today. It is my dream fulfilled.

For the continuing education, inspiration, and the opportunity to consistently provide my colleagues and the public with good, solid, statistical information and well-researched facts, I thank the American Society of Plastic Surgeons (ASPS). I began my involvement with this prestigious society many years ago as the National Chairperson of the Young Plastic Surgeons Committee. Assuming a great number of responsibilities, I became "hooked" on public education. As the years went on, I became a national media spokesperson for ASPS and continue in that role today, often being called upon for interviews and public speaking. My involvement in the American Society for Aesthetic Plastic Surgery (ASAPS) also expands my ability to educate and communicate.

To the many dedicated plastic surgeons, pioneering researchers, and educators who are members of the ASPS and ASAPS, you have my admiration and gratitude for maintaining the highest ethical and educational standards.

I would like to thank the professors at Northwestern Memorial Hospital who painstakingly taught me how to become a plastic surgeon. My special appreciation to Norman Hugo, MD, for bringing me to Northwestern to do my surgical residencies and for getting me involved with ASPS when I first became a member. Thank you also to Peter McKinney, MD, for all his instruction and advice and for bringing me on board with ASAPS. My gratitude as well to B. Herold Griffith, MD, Bruce Bauer, MD, Victor Lewis, MD, John Smith, MD, and in loving memory of Martin Sullivan, MD.

Thank you to my marketing team, Rubin & O'Brien for helping me to increase the public awareness of my practice. I also wish to express my gratitude to James H. Wells, MD, for his encouragement and support of this endeavor.

And last but not least, my sincere appreciation to Marie Kuechel for inviting me to co-author this book and for putting up with my "nit-picking" personality. As a teammate and soul mate, I have only the greatest admiration for her. She approaches life with incredible enthusiasm and efficiency. Anytime I felt stressed by the magnitude of the project, Marie's optimism kept my eye on the prize. It gives me great pride and satisfaction to see my name next to hers on the cover of this extraordinary book. Thank you Marie.

Diane L. Gerber, MD

I am in a constant state of learning. And while every person I encounter in life teaches me something, it is the physicians I work with who have taught me so much about plastic surgery and about integrity. I thank you for your knowledge, patience, and trust. I also thank the consumers of plastic surgery, whose questions, misconceptions and expectations lead us to better understand and communicate the specifics of medical care. You all fuel my fire.

I also extend my thanks to James H. Wells, MD, the first plastic surgeon I worked with at the American Society of Plastic Surgeons in development of public and patient education programs. I am most fortunate that my first experience in working with plastic surgeons was the highest model of excellence and compassion. Dr. Wells, you have set the bar for me, both of what I believe every physician should be, and of what I strive for my contributions to this industry to be. Thank you.

To my co-author, Diane L. Gerber, MD, FACS, who is a most remarkable woman of kindness, energy, and precision, and who I had the privilege to work with twice in the span of a decade: you are a remarkable and inspiring model of excellence. Personally, your compassion, caring, and personal attention to your patients is something that every plastic surgery patient should expect to receive. Professionally you are a master of your specialty. Both professionally and personally, my most sincere thanks.

I also must extend my thanks to David P. Van Dam, MD, James G. Hoehn, MD, Brian J. Kinney, MD, Walter L. Erhardt, Jr., MD, Mark L. Jewell, MD, Foad Nahai, MD, and Joseph J. Disa, MD, for their inspiration and kindness.

In addition, I add my thanks to all my friends at the American Society of Plastic Surgeons and the American Society for Aesthetic Plastic Surgery, namely Karen E. Bresson and Robert and Linda Stanton, respectively. Your dedication to this specialty of medicine and to continuously elevating standards of care and safety is a model for the medical industry, worldwide.

My thanks also to my parents, Victor and Maria, and Andreas and Theresa for helping me in my greatest job in life—caring for my sons Nicky and Andy—while I pursue my profession. And to John, Nicholas, and Andrew—your patience and love is my greatest blessing. Thank you. You are my world, my life, and my every hope.

Marie Czenko Kuechel, MA

Too many questions, straightforward answers

When we hear about, read about, or talk about plastic surgery, the focus is so often only on one-half of the story. In 2003, the American Society of Plastic Surgeons reported nearly 8.8 million aesthetic or appearance enhancing plastic surgery procedures performed by board-certified plastic surgeons in the United States. Also in 2003, ASPS reported just over 6.2 million reconstructive procedures performed by the same group of physicians out of medical need, but still focused on human appearance, form and function.

Consumers and media focus most often on the half of plastic surgery that includes those procedures strictly to improve appearance, be it reversing the signs of aging, or refining what heredity, lifestyles, and our environment may bestow. But what is often forgotten is that both sides of plastic surgery are vital to modern medicine and are most fulfilling experiences for those more than 14 million patients who undergo plastic surgery each year—patients who range in age from newborn babies through the spectrum of life.

This book is about more than just those 8.8 million aesthetic plastic surgery procedures performed each year. It includes what you need to know about plastic surgery to enhance your appearance, and, more importantly, how you identify the credible and appropriate providers of the procedures we commonly classify as plastic surgeons. It also answers your questions about your interest, desires, expectations, and responsibilities as a patient seeking plastic surgery.

As you read this book, don't simply think about plastic surgery as a means for people to improve personal appearance. Know, also, that plastic surgery miraculously restores function—totally or partially—in cases such as:

- a child born with a birth defect
- a trauma victim horribly disfigured
- a burn victim whose flesh has melted away
- a cancer patient who, to save his or her life, must consent to having portions of his or her body excised
- the worker whose fingers no longer function from the repetitive motions that result in carpal tunnel syndrome

All of these cases and more, along with those procedures that make us look younger and more attractive, are what plastic surgery is defined to be. But plastic surgery, including procedures that are not surgical at all, would be nothing without the caring, compassionate, and unbelievably skilled physicians who perform these procedures. Most of these providers are not performing plastic surgery simply to make money from the insecurities of others. Rather, these are medical doctors and surgeons who perform plastic surgery procedures to fulfill those they treat by practicing with dedication, and integrity to their specialty and to their patients.

PART ONE

Plastic Surgery: Definitions and Desire

What is plastic surgery?

Why should I consider having plastic surgery?

Why wouldn't I consider having plastic surgery?

What are realistic expectations?

More . . .

An interest in plastic surgery is not exclusive to only those people who plan on having plastic surgery. Today, so much media and consumer information exists on medical treatments—plastic surgery—that improve appearance and reverse the signs of aging that it is difficult not to be curious. What really is plastic surgery, and why do growing numbers of people undergo what we commonly term "plastic surgery" procedures each year? The answer to both questions is not so simple to define. Plastic surgery has, in some cases, become a generic term for what is a highly specialized field of medicine. And why growing numbers of people undergo aesthetic plastic surgery procedures is hopefully the result of true patient desire, not curiosity.

The information you need to determine why you should or should not consider plastic surgery begins in this book. It may surprise those who are simply curious, will enlighten those considering plastic surgery, and hopefully make us all better-informed consumers about the medical treatments that enhance personal appearance.

1. What is plastic surgery?

Plastic surgery has nothing to do with plastic or plastic products, nor does it imply something that is phony. Plastic surgery is derived from the Greek word "plasticos," which means to fashion or shape.

Plastic surgery is a specialty of modern medicine. It includes both reconstructive and aesthetic procedures of the entire face and body: the skin, fat, muscle, cartilage, and bone. Founded in the late 16th century by the physician Gaspare Tagliacozzi, this medical specialty strives to "bring back, refashion and restore to wholeness the features that nature gave but chance destroyed...not as a mean artifice but as an alleviation of illness." Not until the 20th century did modern plastic surgery begin to take shape with the founding of the American Board of Plastic Surgery in 1937. But it was not until the late 20th century that plastic surgery developed into a term not only for a specialty of medicine, but also for specific types of medical procedures and treatments including reconstructive and aesthetic procedures, and surgical and nonsurgical treatments.

Reconstructive Plastic Surgery

Reconstructive procedures are performed to treat disease, illness, trauma, and birth defects. These procedures are done to restore the human body to "normal" in form and function. Reconstructive plastic surgery includes such things as:

- Removal of tumors
- Breast reconstruction following mastectomy
- Reduction of overly large and painful breasts
- Facial or body reconstruction following cancer
- Cleft-lip and palate surgery
- Restoration and reconstruction of other pediatric anomalies and birth defects, including the separation of conjoined twins
- Carpal tunnel syndrome, rheumatoid arthritis, and other diseases and disorders of the hands
- Trauma to skin, soft tissues, and bones to create an outcome that is aesthetically pleasing and to minimize scarring
- Some forms of scar revision
- Reattachment of severed fingers, toes, and limbs

• Treatment of burns, including reconstruction of severely debilitating and disfiguring burns

Aesthetic Plastic Surgery

Aesthetic plastic surgery encompasses those procedures that are clearly elective and pursued by individuals to enhance appearance. Aesthetic surgery is performed to enhance genetic features or to change conditions that result from the environment and aging. It includes both surgical and nonsurgical (also called noninvasive) techniques.

Plastic Surgery Today

Until 2003, reconstructive and aesthetic procedures each held about an equal share of plastic surgery procedures overall. In 2003 alone, the American Society of Plastic Surgeons (ASPS) reported more than 6.2 million reconstructive procedures done by board-certified plastic surgeons.* In 2003, for the first time, the number of aesthetic procedures reported was significantly greater than reconstructive procedures, with 8.8 million aesthetic procedures reported by ASPS in 2003.

While plastic surgery has grown in consumer demand, it has also evolved to be a generic label for medical appearance-enhancing procedures and treatments. To fill that demand, there are more providers than ever

---

*The term *board-certified* is used throughout this book to define appropriate providers of plastic surgery procedures. This group includes those physicians who are *board-eligible* in a defined specialty. Board-eligible includes those physicians who have successfully completed an American Board of Medical Specialties residency but have not yet completed their exams. In many specialties, a physician must be in practice for a few years before he or she is permitted to take the exams.

offering these treatments. Some providers are doctors who are not board-certified to perform plastic surgery, and in some cases the plastic surgery providers may not even be physicians.

2. What is the difference between plastic, aesthetic, and cosmetic surgery?

Plastic surgery encompasses both reconstructive and aesthetic (cosmetic) procedures. The terms *aesthetic* and *cosmetic* describe only those medical procedures performed to fulfill your desire to improve personal appearance.

But the terms *plastic, aesthetic,* and *cosmetic* are often used interchangeably to describe certain procedures. And they are often used interchangeably to describe the providers of these procedures. Any doctor can technically call him or herself a "plastic surgeon" or a "cosmetic surgeon" if he or she wishes. The true distinction lies in training and board-certification, not the self-imposed title of the person performing that procedure. The American Board of Medical Specialties recognizes only one plastic surgery board: The American Board of Plastic Surgery.

Thus, the term used to label a given procedure—plastic, aesthetic, or cosmetic—is not nearly as important as the credentials and training of the physicians who use these terms. Understanding what defines a credible plastic surgery provider is vital to your enlightenment, safety, and satisfaction with plastic surgery. It is so important that Chapter 2 is devoted to:

• Defining who the appropriate providers of plastic surgery are

- How to recognize these physicians
- Where to verify that a physician is a legitimate provider of specific types of plastic surgery procedures

Read Chapter 2 carefully. The information is vital to identifying which physicians are appropriately trained to perform plastic surgery and which ones are not.

3. Who has plastic surgery?

People who live in Hollywood and wealthy socialites do not comprise the world of plastic surgery patients. Men, women, and children of any age can be plastic surgery patients. According to the American Society of Plastic Surgeons, in 2003 the nearly 8.8 million people who underwent aesthetic plastic surgery procedures performed by a board-certified plastic surgeon included:

- 83% Caucasian patients, 6% Hispanic patients, 5% African-American patients, and 3% Asian-American patients
- 45% adults aged 35 to 50
- 1.35 million men
- 45% who had previous plastic surgery
- 32% who had more than one procedure during a single session

Nose reshaping, liposuction, breast augmentation, and eyelid surgery were the most common surgical procedures. Wrinkle reduction by injection (or Botox® Cosmetic therapy), chemical peel, and microdermabrasion were the most common nonsurgical procedures.

Of the 6.2 million reconstructive procedures performed by board-certified plastic surgeons in 2002, there were:

- 4.46 million tumor-removal patients
- nearly 200,000 hand-surgery patients
- over 100,000 female breast-reduction patients, an increase of more than 150% since 1992
- over 68,000 female breast-reconstruction patients
- nearly 44,000 cases of animal bite injury repair
- nearly 43,000 cases to repair birth defects

4. Why should I consider plastic surgery?

If you have a physical need to restore a more normal appearance and function, then you should consider reconstructive plastic surgery. If you want to enhance what is otherwise considered a normal human feature, then you should consider aesthetic plastic surgery. This includes both procedures that reverse or improve the signs of aging (rejuvenation surgery) and those that enhance appearance.

No one can or should tell you why you should consider plastic surgery for aesthetic reasons. You should be able to clearly define your desire to improve aging or to enhance facial or body appearance. Others may support you in your decision, but the decision to have plastic surgery should be yours alone.

5. Why wouldn't I consider aesthetic plastic surgery?

Asking yourself why you would not or should not consider plastic surgery is as critical as asking why you should consider it.

First, you should not have aesthetic plastic surgery to improve or enhance appearance if you have serious health issues. Take care of your health first.

The American Society of Plastic Surgeons reports that in 2003, 45% of plastic surgery patients seen by their members were repeat patients, not necessarily for the same procedure.

Plastic Surgery: Definitions and Desire

You should not consider plastic surgery if you don't have a personal desire to improve your appearance in some way. While the support of your spouse, partner, family, friends, and your physician is highly desirable, no one should ever bully you into having any surgical procedures.

You should also not consider plastic surgery if your life is in a transition that leaves you vulnerable or searching for dramatic personal change. Plastic surgery will not change your whole life; those who expect that it will do so will be very disappointed. This doesn't mean that plastic surgery is not fulfilling. The outcomes of plastic surgery may give you the new confidence that will allow you to take different directions in your life. It is your motivation, your ambition, and your desire that will make this happen.

Only you can decide your comfort level with plastic surgery. Even if your surgeon does not exclude you from having plastic surgery for health reasons, you should not consider plastic surgery if you are not willing to accept that there is always the potential for risk and complications, even with the most skilled care.

You should not consider plastic surgery unless you have realistic goals for the outcomes and realistic expectations of the process. You must also be willing to accept all the patient responsibilities defined in this book, and specifically those defined by your surgeon, to improve your safety and your chances for favorable outcomes.

6. What are realistic goals?

Realistic goals mean that you fully understand what plastic surgery can and cannot achieve for you. Before you consider plastic surgery and before you make the decision to have plastic surgery, ask yourself the following questions:

- Why do I want to have plastic surgery?
- What do I specifically hope to accomplish through plastic surgery?
- Do others see what I see and what I hope to improve through plastic surgery?
- What is the risk to my health and my life by the treatment necessary to achieve what I want to accomplish, and am I willing to accept this risk?
- What expectation do I have for the physical outcome of plastic surgery?
- What are my expectations concerning my daily life?
- What are the expectations concerning my life overall?
- Is this decision mine alone?
- Do those who support me in my daily life also support my desire for plastic surgery?

If you can answer these questions confidently, you and your surgeon together can determine whether your goals are realistic. Realistic goals are defined as those that are both safe and attainable. In addition, realistic goals for aesthetic plastic surgery are:

- Not extreme
- Not the goals of anyone other than the patient
- Not life-changing
- The goals of emotionally healthy individuals who want to improve their appearance for themselves

7. What are realistic expectations?

Realistic expectations include: (1) a complete understanding of the plastic surgery process and (2) accepting that process as necessary to achieve your realistic goals.

The process of plastic surgery, like any medical treatment or surgery, involves:

• Pretreatment or preoperative patient obligations
• Varying degrees of discomfort, anxiety, and pain
• Time commitment for the procedure and recovery
• Posttreatment or postoperative patient obligations
• Potential for unfulfilled goals and possible undesirable results
• Potential for physical risk
• Financial obligation

The difference between aesthetic plastic surgery and other medical treatments is that you are undergoing treatment by choice. Aesthetic treatment is not performed to promote better health. It includes a personal, emotional, and physical investment. You cannot expect to be fully satisfied by plastic surgery—even if the actual physical outcome was what you expected—unless you are prepared fully for the process that outcome will require.

8. What is a "good candidate"?

Your plastic surgeon should discuss with you whether he or she defines you as a good candidate for a given procedure. A good candidate is not simply someone who is unhappy with an aspect of his or her appearance. A good candidate begins with someone who is unhappy with a real defect in appearance, not a flaw that no one else can see.

This is not a definition of body dysmorphic disorder, a term that has been used to label some plastic surgery patients. Body dysmorphic disorder (BDD) is a very serious psychological condition, a preoccupation with an imagined physical defect or a vastly exaggerated concern about a minimal defect. BDD is similar to obsessive-compulsive disorder. Psychologists note BDD as generally beginning in adolescence. Individuals with BDD are so troubled by the perceived defect that they obsess over it for more than one hour per day. Indeed, someone with BDD is not a good candidate for plastic surgery. BDD should only be diagnosed by a licensed and appropriately trained psychologist or psychiatrist; it is not a label to be used by opponents of plastic surgery.

The definition of a good candidate in plastic surgery is a patient:

- Who would, in fact, achieve an improvement of the areas treated and therefore of his or her overall appearance
- Whose expected outcomes are safely attainable
- Who is in appropriate condition, physically and emotionally, to undergo treatment
- Who is motivated by his or her own desire
- Who fully understands and accepts the process, risk, and patient obligations of plastic surgery
- Who is confident and communicative

Why is a good candidate for plastic surgery someone who is confident and communicative? If you undergo surgery voluntarily and are not confident about your own intentions, your expectations, or the skill of your provider, you may be disappointed with the process and the results. Furthermore, if you do not

In 2001, an exclusive survey conducted by the American Society for Aesthetic Plastic Surgery reported that 2% of individuals who consult with their members exhibit symptoms of BDD. In addition, that same study reported that "84% of ASAPS members refuse to perform surgery on people who display symptoms suggestive of BDD, and 50% of those repsonding have referred such patients for psychiatric consultation."

fully communicate with your provider, he or she will not be able to guess your expectations or risk factors. This situation is also a setup for disappointment or safety issues. A good candidate for plastic surgery has the greatest opportunity for a smooth process and successful outcome.

PART TWO

Plastic Surgery Providers

What defines a qualified plastic surgeon?

What other credentials and factors should be considered?

How can a qualified provider be found?

More . . .

You understand what plastic surgery is and how it specifically applies to your case. Your desire is realistic. Now you need to find a qualified provider with whom to consult. If you are uncertain whether your goals can be fulfilled or how they can be fulfilled, a qualified provider should educate you so that you may make an informed decision. A qualified provider should also define whether or not you are a good candidate by evaluating in you the exact things you have questioned of yourself, as defined in Question 8.

9. Who performs plastic surgery?

Plastic surgery can be performed by any physician regardless of specialty. There are no legislative or legal requirements to restrict physicians from performing certain types of medical procedures, regardless of training or skill. Only state legislation restricts providers from allowing certain medical procedures.

As a potential patient, you must take the initiative to find out whether a particular physician is qualified to perform plastic surgery procedures. Questions to ask include: Is this doctor board-certified in plastic surgery or a specialty related to the procedure I am considering? Does this physician have recognized post-graduate medical training? What credentials has this physician achieved? Does this physician have sub-specialty training, credentials, or certificates? Has this particular doctor performed the procedure that I am interested in? How often? What are the outcomes of the patients treated in the procedure I am considering by this physician? With all of the above information in hand, you can then ask yourself whether this particular doctor is a good candidate to perform a specific procedure on you.

Questions 10 through 13 will help you search for the best possible provider of the right care for you. Remember to always check credentials.

10. What defines a qualified provider?

Qualified providers of plastic surgery procedures are those physicians with board certification that is recognized by nationally and internationally accepted standards. In the United States, the American Board of Medical Specialties (*www.abms.org*) is the umbrella organization of 24 approved medical specialty boards. "The intent of the (ABMS) certification of physicians is to provide assurance to the public that those certified by an ABMS Member Board have successfully completed an approved training program and an evaluation process assessing their ability to provide quality patient care in the specialty." In Canada, board certification is defined and awarded by the Royal College of Physicians & Surgeons of Canada (*www.rcpsc.medical.org*).

Board certification, in many cases, is a very complex and thorough process that takes several years after completion of medical school and includes formal

Action has begun at the state level to introduce legislation about physician advertising and medical education. In 2004, California upheld state legislation that limits physician advertising to content related to one's specialty and limits the use of the term board-certified to specialties approved by the American Board of Medical Specialties or equivalent boards. At the same time, Florida introduced legislation that would require physicians to disclose board certification in advertising and require physicians to specify medical training. This legislation does not preclude the need for consumers to research provider credentials. But it does highlight the importance of board certification and specialization, which are the starting point of choosing a qualified provider in any medical specialty.

Plastic Surgery Providers

resident

a licensed physician, who has completed medical school and is in a post-graduate training program of a given specialty.

training as a **resident** in one or more surgical special-ties. Board-*eligible* providers can be considered quali-fied providers of plastic surgery in the medical specialties defined below who have not yet com-pleted written and oral exams. When you consult with a provider who is not yet board-certified, ask that provider when the board certification is antici-pated. You should also question a provider who has finished training many years previously and is not yet board-certified.

Board-Certified Plastic Surgeons

The ABMS recognizes only one plastic surgery board. That board is The American Board of Plastic Surgery (*www.abplsurg.org*). Those holding ABPS certification are the only physicians to appropriately hold the title of "plastic surgeon." Physicians with board certification in other specialties are not accredited to perform *all* types of plastic surgery procedures of the face and entire body.

Board-Certified Facial Plastic and Reconstructive Surgeons

The specialty of otolaryngology—head and neck sur-gery (ear, nose, throat)—is recognized by the ABMS. Physicians with certification by the American Board of Otolaryngology or with certification by the ABPS may elect to apply for specialty certification by the Ameri-can Board of Facial Plastic and Reconstructive Surgery to qualify them in plastic surgery procedures of the face, head, and neck. The sub-specialty certification of plastic surgery of the head and neck for both board-certified plastic surgeons and board-certified otolaryn-gologists is approved and recognized by the ABMS.

Other Board Certifications

The American Board of Dermatology and the American Board of Ophthalmology are among ABMS member boards. However, there is no sub-specialty board certification specific to plastic surgery related to either of these board certifications. Dermatologists and ophthalmologists are trained in procedures related to their specialties that can be considered plastic surgery. The board-certified dermatologist is trained to perform certain procedures specific to skin and soft tissue, and the ophthalmologist to perform procedures specific to the eyes and surrounding tissue.

As of the writing of this book, only those named above hold ABMS-recognized board certification to perform appropriate plastic surgery procedures. There are, however, other organizations that offer credentials or certification relating to or that include limited plastic surgery procedures. For example, physicians who hold a medical degree in dentistry may elect to undergo an added minimum four-year hospital surgical residency program to qualify in oral and maxillofacial surgery. These physicians may perform reconstructive procedures of the bones and soft tissue of the head and neck that are considered plastic surgery, but they are, by no means qualified in all aspects of plastic surgery.

11. Are these the only credentials to consider?

Checking board certification is a good place to begin when considering treatment by a provider in plastic surgery. In no way is board certification the *only* qualification. Beyond board certification, you should consider a provider's specialized training and experience in performing a given procedure.

Access to information

The following Web sites offer both definitions of board certification and the opportunity for you to confirm a physician's board certification with the related specialty.

American Board of Medical Specialties

www.abms.org

Royal College of Physicians & Surgeons of Canada

www.rcpsc. medicine.org

American Board of Plastic Surgery

www.abplsurg.org

American Board of Otolaryngology

www.aboto.org

American Board of Facial Plastic and Reconstructive Surgery

www.abfprs.org

American Board of Dermatology

www.abderm.org

American Board of Ophthalmology

www.abop.org

Plastic Surgery Providers

Furthermore, even though a procedure may be performed in a physician's office or an outpatient surgical facility, you must make certain that your physician has privileges to perform that same procedure in a local, accredited hospital or full-service medical center. A physician who is on staff and has privileges to perform specific plastic surgery procedures at an accredited hospital has had his or her training and credentials reviewed by that hospital's board of medical specialists before being given privileges.

12. Are there other factors to consider in evaluating a physician?

You should ask about the physician's professional affiliations and appropriate providers of specific treatments. Professional affiliations include, most specifically, the organizations that support the training, education, and research of plastic surgery and of physicians holding appropriate qualifications to perform plastic surgery procedures. In addition, these organizations require certain standards of practice, ethics, and continuing medical education, all with the mission to uphold patient safety.

Board-Certified Plastic Surgeons

For board-certified plastic surgeons, look for membership in the American Society of Plastic Surgeons (ASPS). ASPS requires members to be board-certified by the American Board of Plastic Surgery, and requires added ongoing training and competency (accredited continuing medical education or CME) in plastic surgery procedures each year. The organization also requires members to operate only in surgical facilities that are appropriately licensed or accredited (see Question 28), and to adhere to patient safety standards and ethical standards, which include such things as advertising, patient rights, and privacy.

Board-certified plastic surgeons can belong to sub-specialty groups. For example, those board-certified plastic surgeons practicing aesthetic plastic surgery may belong to the American Society for Aesthetic Plastic Surgery (ASAPS). Those who practice maxillofacial surgery (surgery specializing in the jaws and face region) may belong to the American Society for Maxillofacial Surgeons. Although there are many other sub-specialty groups, the primary professional membership for any board-certified plastic surgeon is the American Society of Plastic Surgeons.

Board-Certified Facial Plastic and Reconstructive Surgeons

For physicians using the title facial plastic surgeon, the professional affiliation to consider is the American Academy of Facial Plastic and Reconstructive Surgeons. Members of the AAFPRS include physicians who are board certified in otolaryngology (ear, nose, throat), plastic surgery, ophthalmology (eyes), and dermatology (skin). Like ASPS (although unrelated), the AAFPRS requires members to adhere to continuing medical education requirements, and safety and ethical standards in practice.

Other Certifications

For the dermatologist, the American Academy of Dermatology and the American Society for Dermatologic Surgery both require members to be certified by the

American Board of Dermatology. In conjunction with these credentials, you should ask about accredited training and competency specific to the procedures of the skin and soft tissue you are considering. For the ophthalmologist, the American Academy of Ophthalmic Plastic Surgery offers membership to board-certified ophthalmologists who have demonstrated added accredited training and competency in plastic surgery procedures limited to the ocular (or eye area) facial region.

In addition to these groups, a physician may have regional society memberships or sub-specialty society memberships that further a physician's recognition among his or her medical peers. The lists of these groups are endless, and while membership to some has great value, what is most relevant to the consumer is primary professional affiliation based upon ABMS-recognized board specialization.

Appropriate Providers

A plastic surgeon certified by the American Board of Plastic Surgery is trained to perform plastic surgery procedures of the entire face and body. Common sense is your greatest guide when considering any other provider of plastic surgery procedures.

Make certain the provider is appropriate for the procedure you planning. For example, a facial plastic surgeon is obviously not one who, by credential, should perform breast surgery. A dermatologist is obviously not one who, by credential, should perform a surgical facelift. An ophthalmologist is one who, by credential, should obviously not perform liposuction. In addition, you should question a provider regarding the number of like procedures he or she has performed, and ask to see his or her patient photographs of outcomes.

Then you may want to do a bit more homework. You can check with your state medical board about the physician's licensing and inquire with the state board of professional regulation about complaints that may have been filed against the physician.

13. How do I find a qualified provider?

Hopefully you won't find your provider by responding to bargain advertisements or special offers. While advertising is a common and acceptable practice, it may not tell you the whole story. Always check credentials.

Internet searches or directories for the procedure you are considering also may be helpful. Among the different directories, first consider those of the medical societies and professional affiliations for physicians qualified to perform plastic surgery procedures. All of these groups have directories or referral services available on the Internet.

There are many other directories, physician finder, and listing services available on the Web. These are commonly subscription services—a physician pays to be listed—and there may be no requirement or screening of credentials. *You* must always check credentials.

Referral

A referral by a trusted physician, family member, or friend is another good first step in finding the right plastic surgeon for you. As in any case, make your final

Plastic Surgery Providers

Physician Web site directories of qualified plastic surgery providers:

The American Society of Plastic Surgeons
www.plastic surgery.org

The American Society for Aesthetic Plastic Surgery
www.surgery.org

The American Academy of Facial Plastic and Reconstructive Surgery
www.aafprs.org

American Academy of Dermatology
www.aad.org

American Society for Dermatologic Surgery
www.aboutskin surgery.org

The American Society of Ophthalmic Plastic and Reconstructive Surgery
www.asoprs.org

selection for a provider based on your research of credentials, affiliations, and the appropriateness of treatment relative to credentials and experience.

Once you have carefully confirmed a provider's board certification, affiliations, training, and experience, check on the licensing or accreditation of the facility where your surgery will be performed. This is discussed thoroughly in Part 5.

PART THREE

Where to Begin

How do I choose a physician to perform my surgery?

What is involved in a consultation?

What is informed consent?

More ...

Once you are ready to explore options in plastic surgery, you need to educate yourself about providers and procedures. The educational process can be very enlightening and fulfilling when you know what to expect and what is expected of you. This is the process of preparing for your consultation or first visit with a plastic surgeon.

14. Where do I begin?

Start with yourself. Try to identify the physical characteristics you feel good about and those you wish to improve.

Your desire for plastic surgery should be specific. You must not expect that plastic surgery will dramatically change your life. True, cases of reconstruction that rebuild and restore features afflicted by trauma, disease, or birth defect can make a significant change in appearance and function. But even these procedures cannot change who you are as a person or change the course of your life. You must be able to accept what plastic surgery can and cannot achieve. Once you have come to a decision, you should feel confident about yourself, your goals to pursue, and the changes you desire.

Conversely, do not undergo plastic surgery to please anyone else. For example, even if your husband expresses a wish that you had bigger breasts, don't undergo surgery for him. If you chose to have plastic surgery, you should do it for yourself.

Plastic surgery is not a simple process. Even when you are confident that you want to have plastic surgery, you need to take the initiative—go out and find the provider and the situation that is right for you. Regardless of qualifications and credentials, providers address patients and cases differently. Take the time to consult with more than one provider. Ask questions about your options and the personal investment in time and money associated with achieving your goals.

Money is a big issue to many people. However, you cannot let money influence your choices for consultation. Complimentary consultations (those free of charge) are offered by many providers. The time and money spent to consult with a physician are minimal compared to the investment of treatment. Consultations are essential to your finding and choosing the right provider. A consultation is your personal window of time with the provider, where you can: (1) review credentials, training, and expertise on the procedure you want to have done; (2) ask relevant questions one-on-one; (3) see photographs of similar procedures for others; and (4) determine whether you are confident in the abilities of the doctor.

15. How do I choose a physician to perform my plastic surgery?

Do not choose your plastic surgeon based on money, emotion, or impulse.

First, conduct your research. Use referrals or directories to find the specialists with appropriate, recognized credentials. Then within that parameter begin your homework:

- Visit that physician's Web site.
- Visit the Web sites of the professional organizations, including hospitals to which the physician belongs.
- Telephone the office of those physicians you are considering. Ask specifically if that physician performs the procedure(s) of interest. Do not expect the

receptionist to answer detailed procedural questions; leave those for your consultation. If you choose to schedule a consultation, ask the office to send you any information relative to your interest and his or her practice. Review all your materials prior to your consultation, and be ready with questions.

• Research again. If you are choosing to undergo plastic surgery, you should take the initiative to be as fully informed as possible. Do your own homework on those treatments and procedures that might be right for you. The Web sites of the plastic surgery professional societies, the same sites you visit to verify credentials (see Questions 10–13), are the best place to obtain consumer information on procedures. These sites specifically offer objective, candid, and valid consumer information that is most likely to be reviewed for consistency and accuracy by leaders in that specialty. For more research, you can visit the Web sites of medical manufacturers and of pharmaceutical companies. For example, if you are considering breast implants, you might visit the manufacturer's Web site for information specifically about the implants recommended for you. Reviewing third-party media (such as the Internet and magazines) can be helpful as long as you pay close attention to detail and are not influenced by other messages often used to attract your interest.

16. What, beyond credentials, should I consider when making a decision on providers?

If your search for the right provider can be considered as a house, credentials are your foundation, experience is your framework, and the individual physician is your shelter. Review again the specific credentials of any provider you consider, and make certain all privileges and credentials are active and in good standing by contacting the state medical licensing board. Ask, "How many times have you done this procedure?" Then find out what kind of experience the provider has specific to the procedure you are considering. A consultation is your opportunity to ask a provider specifically how he or she will address your case. Realize that experience is not always measured in years; it is measured in satisfied patients and in outcomes.

How you gauge experience is by listening, by reviewing, and by asking questions. These questions may include asking the provider how many times he or she has performed the specific procedure you are considering or that is recommended for you. Listen to how a provider speaks and what he or she says when consulting with you:

- Is the doctor confident, clear, and direct?
- Does he or she understand your needs?
- Does the doctor ask about your expectations?
- Does he or she address your needs specifically and offer not only a recommended course of treatment, but also options that might be appropriate?
- Does he or she answer all of your questions directly, in a way that you fully understand?
- Have the physician and the practice staff given you all the information you feel is important to make a decision?
- Have your budgetary concerns been addressed?

Also, review with that provider his or her pre- and post-treatment photographs of similar cases. Ask if these are the best results the surgeon has achieved and ask to see average results. You should feel comfortable asking

Where to Begin

questions about the results in those photographs and how they were achieved.

Your personal experience is also a very important factor in choosing a plastic surgery provider. You should feel welcomed, comfortable, and secure with the staff in your provider's office. You should also be confident that you are safe and will be compassionately cared for.

17. How do I communicate my expectations?

There is no better way to communicate anything than to do so directly. Ask questions when you need more information or do not understand something. Your consultation is the most important time to communicate your goals and expectations, that is, what you want to improve and how you expect it to be accomplished.

Before your consultation, it is helpful to write down any questions you have. Your list should include questions about the procedure you are considering, and about a provider's credentials and experience. In this way, you are less likely to overlook anything. Take this list with you to every consultation. Jot down information that you may wish to review and compare it with subsequent providers. If new questions arise, you should also call the office after your consultation.

Any procedure, even with the very best care and under the very best of circumstances, can result in an outcome that is not fully predictable. Also, any surgical procedure will leave a scar somewhere. While scars can be minimized, hidden, or very carefully placed, they are permanent and are the trade-off to many procedures. Although popular noninvasive procedures like soft tissue fillers and Botox® do not create scars, you do need to repeat these treatments in order to maintain your results. There are always trade-offs you must consider.

Your expectations are not limited to the outcome of plastic surgery, but also include the process. Tell the physician what you are willing to undergo in order to achieve your goals. Although you may be told your expectations are unrealistic, this doesn't mean you cannot continue to pursue plastic surgery. It does mean that you must reevaluate what you are willing to experience and accept to fulfill your desire. You need to know exactly what surgery and recovery entail, including the amount of time you need to recuperate. Make certain you are fully informed about possible complications as well.

18. What should I expect in a consultation?

During your consultation you will meet with your plastic surgeon. Many physicians also have patient counselors or nurses who will guide you through the consultation process and subsequent perioperative (time before and after surgery) course. However, none of these individuals should ever be a substitute for meeting the physician who will be treating you.

Most consultations begin with discussing your medical history, and short- and long-term goals for plastic surgery. You will be asked specifically about what you wish to accomplish, and you will be informed about the treatments that can achieve your goals. You will be given or should ask to see photographic results of your recommended procedure(s).

The consultation process varies from surgeon to surgeon. If the consultation and first visit are combined, you will be examined so that your physician can evaluate your anatomy and physical condition, and determine how to best achieve your goals. Specifics regarding anesthesia, location of procedures, itemized costs, patient obligations, and the recovery process also will be discussed. Photographs may be taken at this time, or once you have decided to proceed with surgery. Then the process of your procedure will be discussed. Following your consultation or in a subsequent visit, orders will be given for lab tests and medications.

In addition, the after-effects or secondary results of your procedure (sequelae) will be discussed. These include things you should expect as a result of the procedure, such as bruising and scars. Your physician should also directly define possible known risks, including unpredictable or unfavorable outcomes and possible complications of the procedure you are considering. Despite a physician's personal safety record with any given procedure, known risks and complications must be fully disclosed. You will then be asked to sign informed consent documents. Read them carefully. Signing these documents means that you fully understand all of the risks as well as benefits of the procedure (see Question 20).

All of the components of a consultation will occur during one or more visits, depending on your case and the physician's customary practices. A nurse or patient coordinator may guide you through the process. But decisions about procedures to be performed will be determined by you and the plastic surgeon.

19. Why are photographs necessary?

Photographs are necessary for the physician's reference. When performing plastic surgery procedures, your surgeon needs to have a baseline of the anatomy of the areas to be treated. The photos are part of your medical record. To compare oneself before and after treatment in photographs taken in the same light, and at the same angle and distance is truly amazing. Before any photograph of you is taken, even for your private patient record, you must sign a release form that specifically defines how and when a physician may use the photographs taken of you. When signing this release, recall how important it was for you to see the actual outcomes of other cases your physician performed. Realize that on the release form, you, too, may be asked to allow your photographs to be used for in-office patient education.

In addition to photographs taken in the physician's office, it is not uncommon for a patient to come into a consultation with a photograph stating, "This is what I want to look like." While bringing in a photograph of Nicole Kidman's nose or Cindy Crawford's lips may be helpful to visually express your goals, there is a caution: Your physician may not be able to meet the ideal of the photograph you present. Very close to this issue is the debate about computer imaging and plastic surgery. Many professional societies have made strong statements against the use of computer imaging in consultation. The reason is simple: Given the nature of human anatomy and the physiology of healing, no result is fully predictable.

A photograph of what you wish your outcome to be, even through computer imaging, can raise false expectations or serve as an implied guarantee. Don't believe for a minute that any physician can guarantee what your outcome will be.

20. What is informed consent?

Informed consent is a legal term, one that began in the 1950s to protect and educate people who volunteered to be the subjects of medical research. These documents were designed to explain:

- What was being researched
- What were the anticipated outcomes
- What were the known risks
- That there was potential for unknown outcomes as risk factors
- That the research subject or patient fully and voluntarily accepted all of the above.

Today "informed consent" is not very different from those earlier years. It is applied to many more situations now than just medical research, however. Informed consent is used with just about every form of medical treatment except those cases that are life-threatening emergencies.

Plastic surgery informed consent is designed to make certain that you fully understand what to expect and that your physician is confident in your understanding. While many patients believe that informed consent is designed to protect the physician from being sued for negligence, no legal document can protect a physician from clear negligence. Make certain you understand all that a procedure or treatment entails and the possible risks and complications defined in an informed consent document before signing.

Informed consent documents should define specifically any injected or implanted substances that may be used in your plastic surgery, such as:

- the brand of and type of breast implant (not necessarily the exact model)
- the brand of pharmaceutical injectable or implanted soft tissue filler, or solid facial implant
- the brand of wrinkle reducer, such as Botox®

Physicians, including plastic surgeons, are continuously solicited by foreign companies to purchase imported, less-expensive substitutes for U.S. FDA-approved medical devices, implants, and pharmaceuticals. While these substances are marketed as like-substitutes, they are not approved by the U.S. FDA, and therefore their quality and safety has not been tested and documented in the United States. The American Society of Plastic Surgeons, in conjunction with the American Society for Aesthetic Plastic Surgery and the American Society for Dermatologic Surgery, each have position statements advising their members against such importation to uphold their professional societies' commitment to patient safety. As a consumer, you must be certain your physician has defined exactly what will be used in your individual treatment, at the time of treatment, and in any repeated treatments.

Where to Begin

PART FOUR

Paying for Plastic Surgery

Will insurance cover plastic surgery costs?

Are there hidden costs?

Can money be saved on a procedure?

More . . .

You have defined your goals for plastic surgery and are confident in your desire to fulfill those goals. You have found a provider for your plastic surgery and are now ready to progress to actually having plastic surgery. Before you proceed, you need to determine how you will pay for treatment.

The emotional cost of plastic surgery can be high, and the monetary cost of plastic surgery can be equally as high. You must be able to accept the cost of plastic surgery with respect to what you can afford.

21. Will insurance cover my plastic surgery?

Insurance will only cover reconstructive procedures, which are those specifically designed to treat disease or trauma, and to restore malformations of the human body to a more normal appearance. Even in these cases (except emergencies) pre-certification is required. Most physicians' offices will assist you with pre-certification, and all will provide you with the documents necessary for coverage if, indeed, your procedure qualifies for coverage.

While most procedures are clearly aesthetic or reconstructive in nature, there are some gray areas. For example, breast reduction is often considered reconstructive and is thereby covered by insurance. However, in some cases, often based on the amount of tissue to be removed, standards for coverage may not be met. Furthermore, different insurance policies may request documentation of previous medical treatments, various measurements, weight loss records, and so forth, before agreeing to cover the procedure. Many HMOs will not cover breast reduction at all. Hence, always get pre-certification for any potentially covered surgery so that you always know where you stand financially.

Procedures that are most commonly aesthetic in nature can qualify for reimbursement. For example, eyelid surgery is reconstructive whereby other conditions, namely drooping of the upper eyelid, impair vision. Botox® therapy may be covered when used to control facial muscle spasms or to achieve symmetry from conditions such as Bell's palsy.

In addition, there are cases where one procedure may have both reconstructive and aesthetic status. For example, a patient having rhinoplasty or nose surgery to correct a breathing impairment may choose at the same time to have aesthetic concerns addressed. Or a patient having correction of a ventral (middle abdominal) hernia may also choose to have excess tissue removed from the abdominal area (a tummy tuck) performed. In these cases, insurance coverage will likely cover the portion of a procedure that is recommended to improve the condition of your health. As always, however, pre-certification is required.

All insurance carriers have specific standards for coverage and specific procedures you must follow in order to obtain coverage. Coverage is never guaranteed, unless you have checked with your insurance carrier, have followed all policy and procedures for pre-certification and reimbursement, and have written approval.

A very important note: Thanks to the efforts of the American Society of Plastic Surgeons, breast reconstruction is required by law to be covered by any insurance carrier in all 50 states of the United States. In addition, those procedures performed on the opposite breast to achieved symmetry are also required, by law, to be covered. These procedures include breast augmentation, breast lift, and breast reduction, which might otherwise be considered aesthetic.

22. What can I do to have my plastic surgery covered by insurance?

Quite simply, follow procedure for pre-certification and reimbursement when you are having plastic surgery that is entitled to insurance coverage. You cannot do anything to have a purely aesthetic procedure covered by insurance. That would be fraud, and no credible provider will assist you in filing false insurance claims.

23. What will plastic surgery cost?

Your financial obligations will depend on the procedure planned, your geographic region, your surgeon's fees, and where the procedure will be performed. All secondary costs should be clearly defined to you in the process of informed consent. You will be given a specific breakdown of the cost of any procedure based on surgeon's fees, surgical facility fees, the fees for anesthesia, and fees for special medical devices (such as special post-surgical garments). You may also need to pay for preoperative lab work, although lab work may be covered by your insurance.

Most physicians include the cost of follow-up visits in the surgical fees. However, you should still ask specifically if these visits are included.

If you choose to recover in a special postoperative recovery facility, the cost of this, too, should be specifically itemized. This includes everything from your

Some organizations publish "average costs" for specific plastic surgery procedures. Be careful when using this information. In most cases, these dollar amounts are a statement of average surgeons' fees only and do not include the cost of anesthesia, operating facilities, supplies, and pharmaceuticals.

room and board to basic care, amenities, and added services that make your stay more comfortable. These services are your choice, and you have the right to know upfront what those costs will be.

24. What are the hidden costs?

There should be no hidden costs to plastic surgery. All costs, including an estimate of anesthesia fees, should be defined prior to surgery. However, anesthesia fees are often based on time in the operating room and sometimes in the recovery room. These times cannot be precisely determined preoperatively. These are not unexpected, but must be an estimated cost. There may be, however, unexpected costs.

Similarly, just like any medical treatment, the outcomes of plastic surgery are not always predictable. Secondary procedures may be necessary to better achieve your desired outcomes. These are not hidden costs. Accepting the cost of any secondary procedure, one that is not reconstructive in nature, is part of the risk you take in choosing to undergo any elective medical treatment.

In the event of a complication related to your plastic surgery that requires emergency treatment, you may be responsible for the cost of that care. Postoperative emergencies requiring surgery or hospitalization are not likely. However, the potential for serious complications or secondary procedures should be discussed during the informed consent process.

25. How will I pay for plastic surgery?

How you will pay for plastic surgery is entirely your decision. You may choose to finance your procedure if you do not have the cash available to pay for it. Some providers accept credit cards, others may offer financing programs, which may be endorsed or offered through a medical association. Or, you may wish to investigate independent sources of financing. Do not finance anything, plastic surgery or otherwise, if you truly cannot afford it.

If you decide to undergo plastic surgery, be confident about your decision and about your chosen date before scheduling. All providers will require a deposit before surgery, and few will refund this deposit after a certain date if surgery is cancelled for anything other than emergencies. This may seem extreme. But when you make the decision to have plastic surgery, a surgical facility and appropriate staff are reserved for your case on the date and time you have scheduled. Your surgeon has reserved this time exclusively for you, and additional services such as anesthesia may be contracted for your case. In addition, special medical supplies may need to be ordered for which the physician must pay in advance.

No matter whether you must finance plastic surgery or you have the cash on hand to pay for your procedure, make certain that you feel it is worth the cost. To spend several thousand dollars on a surgical procedure you are not fully convinced you want to undergo is truly foolish. You cannot return the procedure, and you cannot get your money back.

26. How can I save money on plastic surgery?

You want a procedure, have researched it thoroughly, and are confident in your choice of a provider. However, the price for the procedure and perioperative care seems too expensive. Do not be afraid to stop and reconsider your decision.

There may be alternative treatments that cost less than what the physician specifically recommends to achieve your goals. For example, a brow lift and face lift may restore your aging face to a more youthful appearance. But if you choose not to pay for those procedures, Botox® therapy and injections of fillers might be a less expensive alternative. Botox can soften brow furrows and creases, and soft-tissue fillers will plump wrinkles to give a more youthful appearance. However, these alternatives cannot mimic the results of a brow lift or face lift. These procedures also have to be repeated later to maintain the results. Thus, while less expensive now, over time you may invest much more money than the original surgery would have cost. When reviewing your alternatives, always weigh the costs in time and money over the long term.

If you have consulted with two plastic surgeons who have board certification and other qualifications, and you are equally impressed with both physicians, of course price is a consideration. However, it is very risky to consider a provider who is not board certified or qualified in the particular procedure you are interested in, or to consider any physician simply on the basis of the cheaper price. You must consider that there is an increased potential for an unsatisfactory outcome and a greater risk to your safety.

One way to legitimately save on plastic surgery is to recover at home instead of a luxurious spa-like facility. Patients can recover safely at home following most plastic surgery procedures with the support of a responsible adult family member, friend, or other caregiver.

PART FIVE

Plastic Surgery and Safety

Where will plastic surgery be performed?

What are the risks of plastic surgery?

What can I do to reduce chances of complications?

What are my responsibilities as a patient?

More . . .

Your decision to undergo plastic surgery must include an evaluation and direct discussion about possible risks and your safety. This discussion is something you must have face-to-face with the physician who is going to treat you. You also must be knowledgeable about the facility in which a procedure will be performed.

Any medical treatment carries some element of risk, including treatment complications, reactions to medications, or unpredictable outcomes. Medicine is not an exact science, and no two people are exactly alike. Your greatest advantage to minimizing risk and complications lies in your choice in providers of plastic surgery, your level of preoperative information, and your compliance with all instructions.

27. Where is plastic surgery performed?

Plastic surgery can be performed in any number of places.

In 2003, the American Society of Plastic Surgeons reports 56% of all aesthetic procedures were performed in office-based surgical facilities; 28% in a hospital setting, and 16% in freestanding surgical facilities.

Noninvasive procedures are most commonly performed in a physician's office examination room. These procedures are not surgical in nature. They include injection therapies and skin rejuvenation procedures such as chemical peels and some laser treatments.

Invasive surgical procedures can be performed in an outpatient setting. Minor procedures, such as excision of skin lesions and scar revisions, may be performed in your doctor's office. More invasive procedures should be performed in a hospital or ambulatory surgical facility. An ambulatory surgical facility is an office-based or freestanding surgical setting. Any facility where invasive surgical procedures are performed must be fully accredited by a nationally recognized organization and/or be state licensed. This is essential to your safety.

28. What is facility accreditation?

A physician must pass written and oral examinations to be board-certified. Likewise, a facility must adhere to very specific requirements for architecture, medical equipment, procedural protocols, and then inspection to be granted accreditation. The following are accepted accrediting organizations for surgical facilities in the United States.

- The American Association for Accreditation of Ambulatory Surgery Facilities (AAAASF); *www.aaaasf.org*
- The Accreditation Association for Ambulatory Health Care (AAAHC); *www.aaahc.org*
- The Joint Commission on Accreditation of Health-care Organizations (JCAHO); *www.jcaho.org*
- Certification to participate in Medicare under Title XVIII
- A state license to operate a medical facility, where required by state law

The Web sites of each of these organizations will give you specific requirements for accreditation and allow you to confirm the accreditation of a facility your physician recommends. In general, these standards include:

- That surgery be performed only by board-eligible or board-certified physicians of the American Board of Medical Specialties (ABMS) holding privileges to perform the same procedures at a local, accredited hospital.
- Anesthesia be administered by only a board-eligible or board-certified anesthesiologist (physician) or certified nurse anesthetist (CRNA).

Plastic Surgery and Safety

- Requirements for staff certification, namely surgical technicians, registered nurses, and licensed practical nurses, including training in advanced cardiac life support.
- The use of advanced monitoring during surgery and immediate recovery.

Furthermore, accreditation requires that a facility adhere to all local, state, and national regulations including sanitation, fire safety, and building codes. It also requires that the facility meet federal laws and OSHA regulations including those for blood-borne pathogens and hazardous waste standards.

In addition to national, voluntary accreditation by the AAAASF, the AAAHC, and the JCAHO, some states require specific certification of facilities participating in Medicare billing. Accreditation is not always a substitute for state licensing of a surgical facility. Some states require licensing and others do not.

In an effort to uphold the highest standards of safety for plastic surgery patients, beginning July 1, 2002, the American Society of Plastic Surgeons (ASPS) and American Society for Aesthetic Plastic Surgery (ASAPS) mandated all of their members to operate in a hospital, or state-licensed or accredited facility. As of the writing of this book, these are the only two organizations imposing this standard.

29. What are the risks of plastic surgery?

The risks of plastic surgery begin with those of any surgical procedure: bleeding, infection, pulmonary emboli, anesthesia complications, and unexpected complications related to individual procedures.

Bleeding: Bleeding externally or under the skin (hematoma) can occur with any surgical procedure and can cause major problems. High blood pressure and medications (such as aspirin, ibuprofen, and some herbal supplements) can cause abnormal bleeding. Your surgeon may ask for certain lab work to check your clotting ability. Some people have genetic bleeding disorders without a previous diagnosis. Again, you must tell your surgeon about all of your medications and bleeding history. If you have accidentally taken a medication that causes bleeding in the few weeks before surgery, notify your surgeon. (See Question 32 for a full explanation on avoiding certain medications.)

Infection: Infection is possible with every surgery, even though strict sterile procedure is followed. You may unknowingly have an infection in your body or reduced ability to fight airborne infections. Again, giving your full health history is imperative. Not all infection, however, is the result of surgery. In fact, infection can present long after surgery, during the healing process. Closely following your surgeon's instructions will not only help to avoid the risk of infection, but it will allow him or her to diagnose it early, when it is more easily controlled.

Embolism: Blood clots that can develop in the legs during or after surgery are among the most serious complications that can occur with surgery of any kind. These clots can lead to pulmonary embolism (blockage of a lung artery) and can be fatal. Careful patient selection through an evaluation of current health and use of medications and supplements, smoking habits, health history, and family health history can help to identify patients who are at greater risk. Specific measures may be recommended to minimize the risk of blood clots, or you or your surgeon may decide the risks of surgery are too great and choose not to undergo surgery. You can help to ensure your own safety by fully disclosing health history and following all instructions you are given.

For long procedures, compression wraps, such as TED stockings or intermittent compression boots, should be used to help prevent emboli. Ask if your surgeon uses any form of compression.

Anesthesia: Anesthetic reactions can range from mild discomfort or irritation at a local anesthetic site to heart arrhythmia and even death. Contemporary anesthesia equipment, however, has made surgery with sedation and general anesthesia much safer than in the past. If your surgery is performed in an accredited freestanding facility, this equipment will have regular inspections to ensure that they are working perfectly. Furthermore, there will be a protocol for immediate transfer to the nearest hospital if there is any serious problem.

Procedural outcomes: Risks related to procedural outcomes will be specifically addressed in definitions of all treatments within this book. What you must understand is that the risk of embolism, infection, or those risks related to anesthesia are no greater for plastic surgery patients than for any patient undergoing elective surgery.

Overall risk

Statistics on mortality demonstrate that surgery in an accredited freestanding facility is as safe as a hospital. Based on a study conducted in 1997 by an independent group of physicians affiliated with the AAAASF and reported in the medical journal *Plastic and Reconstructive Surgery*:

- The rate of serious complications of plastic surgery procedures performed in accredited surgical facilities was less than one half of one percent (0.5%).
- The mortality rate was 1 in 57,000 cases.
- Infection was reported in 0.074% of cases.

Patients required transfer to a hospital in 0.12% of cases.

Healthy people have fewer complications. One of the most important considerations in your safety during plastic surgery is to fully disclose your health history. In addition, you should have your health history fully evaluated by a qualified provider.

30. Why will I need a physical, blood work, or pre-surgical testing?

If you are to have a surgical procedure requiring intravenous or general anesthesia, you will be required to undergo pre-surgical diagnostic testing. These tests are performed to detect possible health or bleeding problems and may be covered by your insurance.

Diagnostic testing may include:

- Blood count (CBC), blood chemistry, blood clotting tests, and possible screening for infectious diseases (such as hepatitis and HIV)
- A pregnancy test
- A chest x-ray and electrocardiogram (ECG) after a certain age, or if there is any preexisting heart or lung disease
- A mammogram for most women above age 30 who are undergoing breast surgery. (For women having breast implants for augmentation, a baseline mammogram is an important point of reference for future comparisons.)

Plastic Surgery and Safety

In addition, patients with known medical problems or those beyond a certain age may require a report, from an internist or general practitioner, giving medical clearance for surgery.

Don't look upon diagnostic testing as a nuisance or unnecessary expense. Medical testing gives your plastic surgeon the assurance that he or she is not causing you harm by proceeding with surgery. In addition, the lab work may identify otherwise unknown, underlying medical problems that are readily treatable when caught early (such as high cholesterol).

31. What can I do to reduce my chance of complications?

Choosing a qualified provider and an accredited surgical facility reduces your chance of complications. But you, too, have obligations as a patient. Your obligations as a plastic surgery patient will be carefully defined by your physician and include, but are not limited to:

- Correctly and fully disclosing and chronic or mild ongoing illness or medical condition, such as urinary tract infection (UTI) or skin rashes.
- Correctly and fully disclosing your health history and that of your immediate family.
- Correctly and fully disclosing aspects of your lifestyle, such as smoking and alcohol consumption, the use of prescriptive and other drugs, the use of vitamins and herbal supplements.
- Listening carefully as instructions and the signs of complications are defined to you.
- Following instructions for preoperative restrictions and purchases, diagnostic tests, etc.

- Disclosing any unexpected illness, fever, skin condition, or other symptoms that develop prior to surgery. These may require that surgery be delayed.
- Reading, understanding, and following instructions for wound care, restrictions, medications, etc.
- Understanding all information regarding complications before your procedure so that you know what to look for and when to call your surgeon afterward.
- Recognizing and reporting any serious problems to your physician as soon as possible.
- Attending all preoperative and postoperative appointments as scheduled.

A good *candidate* for plastic surgery is one who is motivated by his or her own desire, who has realistic expectations, and is in good health. What makes you a good *patient* means accepting responsibility for your health and safety. You must follow your physician's instructions precisely and inform your physician immediately if you develop any health problems either before or after your surgery.

32. Why am I told not to smoke or to avoid certain vitamins and medications?

Some substances interfere with the surgical or healing process. Before the surgical procedure, you will have to stop smoking and quit taking certain medications or vitamins (with your physician's approval).

Smoking: Human cells need oxygen to survive and reproduce, both of which are necessary factors in wound healing. Smoking reduces the amount of usable oxygen in the blood and constricts the vessels so that less blood is brought to the cells. With surgery, the number of vessels delivering blood to the wound is already reduced. Therefore, with smoking and surgery together, some cells are greatly deprived of oxygen and they die. The result is tissue that does not heal, infection, and large, unsightly scars. Furthermore, smoking diminishes lung capacity, and if you are to have sedation or general anesthesia, you may end up with severe respiratory problems, including pneumonia.

Therefore, you will need to quit smoking several weeks prior to any surgical procedure and for several weeks afterward. If you are unable to quit smoking on your own, either get help or cancel the surgery.

Medications: Your plastic surgeon most likely will give you a list of medications to avoid before surgery. If some of them are prescriptions, your prescribing physician will need to give permission for you to stop taking these medications. He or she may also need to give you medical clearance before surgery.

33. Can I choose where my procedure will be performed?

Generally, your plastic surgeon will have a preference as to where your surgery will be performed. If you are given a choice and safety is not an issue, then be sure you know the relative costs.

Recovery choices: There are generally more options given to you with regard to recovery. Today, few procedures require an overnight hospital stay. In most cases, you can recover comfortably at home or in a hotel with assistance from a friend, family member, or hired professional.

Your surgeon may recommend a postoperative care facility that he or she feels is safe and expedient. Here you can recover in a setting that may be comfortable and private with some nursing care. It is always a good idea to visit the facility ahead of time and question the services, amenities, and costs. Then make your decision, based, of course, on your surgeon's recommendation.

34. What type of anesthesia will be used?

The types of anesthesia used in plastic surgery depend upon the depth and extent of surgery and on your health. Your plastic surgeon will give a recommendation, and for some procedures there may be options available to you. Or the anesthesiologist or nurse anesthetist may make recommendations. You should also know the credentials of the person providing anesthesia. That person should be an anesthesiologist (medical doctor) or a CRNA (certified registered nurse anesthetist).

The types of anesthesia used in plastic surgery include:

- Oral
- Topical (cream and gel)
- Injectable (local or regional)
- IV sedation (used with injectable anesthetics)
- General (with or without a tube in your trachea)

Your anesthesia options should be discussed with your plastic surgeon prior to surgery.

35. Can I choose what type of anesthesia will be used?

Your plastic surgeon may give you some choices for anesthesia depending upon the procedure to be performed. For example, some procedures may be performed with general anesthesia or with local anesthesia and IV sedation (such as face lifts), and you may have a choice of anesthesia in these cases. However, if your surgeon has a strong preference for one or the other, the anesthesia with which he or she is most comfortable should generally be used.

Other procedures are commonly performed with local anesthesia alone. But if you are anxious about surgery, you can ask to have Valium or other oral calming medication beforehand. If you are afraid of needles and are scheduling a minor local procedure, you can also ask for a numbing cream prior to any injections.

PART SIX

The Basics of Plastic Surgery

What are wound closure and tissue repositioning?

Is removal of a skin lesion plastic surgery?

How can plastic surgery treat skin cancer?

Can scars be removed or erased?

More . . .

All plastic surgery (other than nonsurgical treatments) involves making cuts (excisions) and closing of the subsequent wounds. Wounds may be caused by external trauma such as lacerations or burns, or by surgery. Additionally, wounds may involve only the skin, or they may affect many layers of tissue.

To understand how plastic surgery can achieve your goals, it is important to know a little about how wounds can be closed. The special techniques of wound closure are the basics for all aspects of plastic surgery, and what you learn in this chapter is essential to understanding the specifics of nearly all plastic surgery procedures.

36. What are wound closure and tissue repositioning?

Some wounds may heal by themselves with appropriate wound care, such as a superficial cut treated with a topical antiseptic. More severe wounds can be treated as follows:

- Simple closure of skin only, using glue, adhesives, and/or sutures.
- Layered closure that includes skin and underlying tissue, using permanent or absorbable internal sutures, possibly with external sutures (uniting two surfaces by sewing), glue, or adhesives.
- A flap of tissue composed of skin and fat, one section of which remains attached to part of its original blood supply while the rest of it is moved to a different location to cover a wound.
- A graft, which is tissue that is completely separated from its blood supply and then placed on or in a defect.

Flaps: When a wound is too large to be closed primarily (simple or layered closure) or when the direction needs to be changed (to achieve the best position of a scar), new tissue needs to be brought to the defect (wound). Flaps provide that tissue, along with a new blood supply that will merge with the surrounding healthy tissue.

There are many kinds of flaps based on location and blood supply:

- A local flap is healthy tissue (skin and fat) next to a wound that is moved to cover the defect. Examples include special incisional techniques such as Z-plasty, W-plasty, or a V-Y advancement flap. (These flaps are named for the shape of the ensuing scar.)
- A distant flap is one of healthy tissue further away from a wound that is moved over or under intervening tissue to cover a defect. An example might be a flap that is taken from the forehead to cover a nasal tip wound.
- A free flap is healthy tissue even further from a wound that has feeding vessels that can be attached to similar vessels adjacent to the wound. Free flaps require specialized microsurgical techniques to connect those vessels (and nerves). An example would be a buttock flap used to reconstruct a breast.
- A composite flap is composed of skin and fat like the other flaps, but it also includes deeper tissues such as muscle or cartilage. The most common type used is a musculocutaneous flap in which most of the flap's blood supply comes from the vessels that feed the muscle. This type of flap can be local, distant, or free. Back and abdominal musculocutaneous flaps also may be used in breast reconstruction.

Grafts: A graft is tissue completely separated from its blood supply that is used to cover or fill a defect. A graft receives its blood supply from surrounding and underlying tissue in its new location. In some cases, flaps may be used in conjunction with grafts to bring in a new blood supply. Grafts are best identified by the type of tissue that is used:

- Skin grafts of partial- or full-thickness skin can be placed on an open wound if the base of the wound is red and healthy.
- Soft tissue grafts using tissues under the skin can be used to fill in soft tissue defects. One's own fascia (the layer of tissue covering the muscles) and fat are frequently used as soft tissue grafts.
- Cartilage grafts can be taken from various locations (such as the nose, ear, or rib) to provide firmer filling. An example is enhancement of a nasal tip using nasal septal or ear cartilage.
- Bone grafts can be taken from various areas (the hip, outer skull, or rib) to provide stronger support to a given area. They are sometimes used to reconstruct or enhance facial structures.
- Composite grafts contain two or more types of tissue and can be used where a thicker fill is required, or to fill in soft tissue and supporting structures. An example would be skin and cartilage taken from the ear to replace a portion of the nose removed in cancer surgery.

Synthetic substances can be used in place of grafts in some cases. Because these substances do not originate from your own body, they are referred to as implants, not grafts. Facial implants, and injected or implanted soft tissue fillers, are fully discussed in the following chapters.

Primary closure, flaps, and/or grafts will be used in all the procedures discussed in the following chapters of this book. For example, a facelift requires flaps of skin and underlying tissue. Breast reduction requires local flaps of skin and distant flaps to reposition the nipple and areola. Wounds are then closed by simple or layered primary closure. By understanding the concepts of wound closure and tissue repositioning, you will be better able to appreciate how plastic surgery works to achieve your goals.

When discussing surgical wounds and how they are closed, it is easiest to begin with the treatment of skin lesions and scars. In both situations, a wound may be created by "excision" that then requires closure.

37. What is a skin lesion or scar, and how is it treated with plastic surgery?

A skin lesion is a nonspecific term used to describe an abnormal area of the skin such as a tumor, wart, cyst, or pigmented area. Skin lesions can be classified into one of the following categories, based on clinical and/or microscopic evaluation:

* Benign: a lesion that has no abnormal cells, such as a cyst, mole, or lipoma (a tumor of fatty tissue).
* Premalignant: a lesion that is still considered to be benign, yet has some atypical (not quite normal) cells. If left alone, this kind of lesion most likely would become malignant (cancerous) at some time.

In 2003, wound care techniques in plastic surgery were used to treat nearly 500,000 cases of laceration repair, animal bite repair, and burn treatment collectively, as reported by the American Society of Plastic Surgeons.

The Basics of Plastic Surgery

Examples include actinic keratosis (a red, scaly lesion caused by sun exposure) and dysplastic nevus (pre-malignant mole).

- Malignant: a lesion that has cancerous cells. Cancerous cells are abnormal cells that replace normal cells, invading and destroying local areas, and sometimes invading other organs of the body.

Malignant lesions of the skin include:

- Basal cell carcinoma: The mildest and most common skin cancer. These may spread and destroy local tissue, but rarely metastasize (spread to distant sites).
- Squamous cell carcinoma: This form of skin cancer spreads locally more quickly and can metastasize.
- Melanoma: Highly malignant. This is the most dangerous form of skin cancer and will metastasize if not treated early.

How it's done: Benign and pre-cancerous lesions

Lesions that are benign are generally harmless to one's health. However, they can be unsightly or uncomfortable. Some benign lesions may simply disappear or may be removed by your own immune system. However, any lesion that has the potential for becoming malignant (pre-cancerous) should be treated more aggressively. If a lesion is simply unsightly, or if it is changing, you may be advised to have it removed. One or more of the following treatments may be used:

- Topical: creams may ablate (remove or destroy the function of) certain benign and precancerous lesions
- Destruction: burning, laser, or cryotherapy (use of cold in treatment)

- Excision with primary repair: simple or layered closure
- Excision with complicated repair: flaps and/or grafts

What you need to know

A potentially malignant lesion is one that must be examined and treated by a board-certified plastic surgeon, facial plastic surgeon, or dermatologist experienced in the diagnosis and treatment of skin cancer. A potentially malignant lesion may have:

- Crusts and does not heal
- A change in appearance, color, texture, or size
- Discomfort

A common approach to identifying a lesion that should be further examined by a physician is referred to as the "ABCs of skin cancer":

- **A:** Asymmetry, where one half of the lesion does not match the other.
- **B:** Border, where the edges of the growth are irregular, notched, or blurred.
- **C:** Color of the growth is not uniform, especially if red, black, or blue is present. Shades of tan, brown, and black are present.
- **D:** Diameter, or a lesion width greater than 6 millimeters (about the size of a pencil eraser) or any new growth of a lesion that was previously stable.

If you have any concern or question about a lesion of any kind, it is important to consult with a qualified physician as soon as possible for proper treatment.

Your obligations

The successful outcome of treating any lesion requires that you follow all of your plastic surgeon's instructions for postoperative wound care. This may include cleansing, the use of ointments, and avoiding sun exposure. Later you may need silicone gel or sheeting to help prevent thickening of your scars.

Your goals

Nearly 4.5 million cases of tumor removal, including tumors of the skin, were reported by the American Society of Plastic Surgeons in 2003.

Your goals for the outcomes of lesion removal can be as varied as the type, size, and location of the lesion itself. However, any type of lesion removal requires creating a wound, and wounds leave scars. While these can be inconspicuous in many cases, there is always the potential that a visible scar will result.

38. How is skin cancer treated?

Board-certified plastic surgeons, facial plastic surgeons, and dermatologists are trained to clinically identify those growths that have a greater likelihood of being skin cancer. However, the only way to accurately determine whether a cancer is present is to remove a portion or all of the skin growth (biopsy) and have the tissue examined under a microscope (usually by a pathologist).

Are you covered?

Skin cancer can be treated a number of ways, and the treatment is usually covered (in part or totally) by medical insurance. Some insurers require preapproval for more complex surgical removal (such as Moh's surgery, described on the next page) or for excision with complex reconstruction. The appropriate treatment choices for skin cancer are determined by the type of cancer and its size and location. These choices should be discussed with your physician.

How it's done

Skin cancer can be treated with several different treatments, depending upon the type, location, and severity.

Early superficial, noninvasive cancers may be treated with:

- Topical chemotherapy creams
- Various ablative techniques using a scalpel, cautery, laser, or cryosurgery. Cyrosurgery freezes the cancerous skin lesion and surrounding tissue. The cancerous cells then die and are naturally shed. This form of treatment is common for some basal cell cancers as well as superficial squamous (not invading deeper tissue) cell cancers. Alternatives to cyrosurgery are to ablate (remove) the skin cancer by scraping or fulguration (scraping with an accompanying electrical or chemical burning to seal blood vessels).
- Excision and wound closure—that is, simple, layered flaps or grafts.
- Moh's surgery is a procedure generally used for cancers whose borders are poorly defined or that occur in locations where every millimeter counts (such as cancers on the eyelids or nose). With this technique, tissue is removed layer-by-layer and examined under a microscope at each stage. Moh's treatment allows a physician to remove the diseased tissue at the surface and to identify where cancerous

The Basics of Plastic Surgery

Skin cancer is the most common form of cancer worldwide. The American Society for Dermatologic Surgery reported over 1.6 million skin cancer treatments by their members in 2003.

An entire book has been written about the treatment of skin cancer and is part of the series of books to which this book belongs. To find out more about skin cancer diagnosis, treatment, and prevention, ask your doctor about 100 Questions & Answers About Skin Cancer, *or visit* www. jbpub.com *to obtain more information about the book.*

cells exist in underlying tissues. It presents two advantages: First, there is a greater likelihood that all the cancerous cells are removed and, therefore, results in a higher incidence of cure. Second, the least amount of healthy tissue is removed so that reconstruction can result in a more aesthetically pleasing outcome. Frozen section diagnosis is a similar technique to Moh's, though not as accurate in poorly defined tumors.

There are cases where removal of skin cancer results in a highly disfiguring wound. In some cases, significant portions of the facial structures can be affected, including the cartilage of the nose or ears. These cases will either have excision and reconstruction in the same procedure, or reconstruction at a later time.

The reconstruction of a wound after excision of skin cancer is as individualized as any plastic surgery treatment. The various techniques of wound closure may be

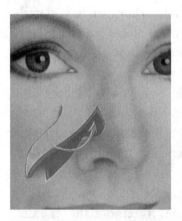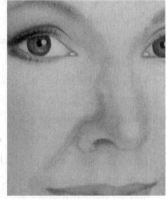

Figure 1 A local flap to reconstruct a skin cancer defect. This is an artist's rendering and does not represent actual patient results. Individual results may vary. Courtesy of the American Society of Plastic Surgeons®. All rights reserved. Learn more at *www.plasticsurgery.org*.

used alone or in combination, and two or more stages (treatments with an interval of time between them) may be required. If you require any advanced form of skin cancer treatment such as Moh's micrographic surgery or reconstruction following treatment, be certain that the surgeon you choose is a board-certified plastic surgeon, facial plastic surgeon, or dermatologist who has expertise in treating skin cancer and in specialized reconstructive techniques. In some cases, different providers may work as a team. For example, with Moh's surgery, a dermatologic surgeon will generally remove the tumor and a plastic surgeon will reconstruct the wound.

The American College of Moh's Micrographic Surgery maintains a listing of active fellows (physicians in post-residency training) who have successfully completed a certified fellowship in Moh's surgery. Visit them at *www.mohscollege.org.*

39. Can scars be removed or erased?

Scar revision is plastic surgery to improve the appearance of undesirable or disfiguring scars. While scar revision can make a dramatic improvement in the appearance and condition of scars, no scar can be completely erased.

Scar revision can be performed on almost any scar, including those that are indented, raised, red, itching, puckering, or constricting. Scar revision is best performed by a board-certified plastic surgeon, a facial plastic surgeon, or in some cases by a dermatologist or general surgeon. In most cases it is a simple office-based, outpatient procedure. However, very large scars, such as those from burns and other serious trauma, may need grafting and/or flap techniques that require hospitalization.

Are you covered?

Some scar revision procedures may be considered recon-structive and thereby are eligible for insurance coverage. Check in advance with your insurance provider.

Good candidates

Scar revision procedures can be performed on any healthy individual. Patients with active skin disease or certain autoimmune disorders may have an impaired healing ability that can affect outcomes. In addition, different skin types produce different scars. Therefore, your skin type and color may determine the type of scar revision procedure recommended for you.

How it's done

Scar revision can be performed using a variety of techniques and treatments. Treatments may be staged or used in combination.

Topical treatments: Silicone sheeting and special tapes, ointments, and gels can be used to improve the appearance and texture of newly formed scars. Silicone sheeting and tapes compress the scar and hold in moisture. Thick scars thus may be reduced or even prevented. In addition, these tapes and gels can refine the color and texture of scars to more closely match surrounding healthy skin.

Injection therapies: Injecting various forms of corti-sone may flatten a raised, firm scar. Injectable fillers can improve the condition of recessed scars or depressions of the skin (see Question 83).

Skin resurfacing: This technique can improve the appearance of mild acne scars and other surface scars. Ablative lasers, chemical peels, and dermabrasion are generally effective for scars that are mildly raised or depressed from the skin surface. Read the specific questions about each of these procedures in Part 11 for more information.

Excision of scars: Excision means cutting out scar tissue. The wound can then be repaired in one or more layers. If the direction of the scar needs to be changed or if healthy skin is not available for direct repair, then flap procedures or skin grafts may be required, as discussed in Question 36. If there is not sufficient tissue available for flap coverage of the wound, a staged procedure using tissue expansion may be necessary. Tissue expansion is a technique that can produce healthy skin near the site of the scar before excision. Tissue expansion surgically places a balloon-like device under the skin with a small valve near the surface of the skin. Over time and multiple visits to your plastic surgeon, the balloon will be filled with sterile liquid. This will stretch and increase the overlying tissue. Once ample tissue is available, the scar can be excised with either a direct or flap closure from the nearby healthy tissue that has been expanded.

What you need to know

Each technique in scar revision carries its own set of complications. All forms of scar revision have the potential to result in a scar that may not be much improved from the original scar. Also, more than one procedure may be necessary.

Your obligations

Follow all of your physician's instructions, particularly with regard to lifestyle issues such as smoking and sun exposure, for the best outcome of your scar revision. While it may be tedious or cumbersome to wear the compression sheeting or tapes and to remember to apply gels as directed, these do influence the outcome of your scar revision.

Your goals

Scar revision is generally permanent, and scars usually improve with time and aging. The one exception occurs in patients who form true "keloids." These are very large, thick scars that invade surrounding tissue and can become worse with time. Keloids may not respond well to any treatment and are more common in darker complexions, such as African–Americans or Asians.

Also, with any new scar, sun exposure can cause abnormal pigmentation that may be permanent. Scar revision can be a relatively simple or complex procedure depending on the size, form, and location of your scar. And even though scar revision may be a minor procedure, it is generally a procedure with high patient satisfaction.

In 2003, the American Society of Plastic Surgeons reported over 232,000 scar revision procedures classified as reconstructive. Additional cases of injectable fillers and resurfacing techniques to improve scars for aesthetic reasons are not included in these numbers.

PART SEVEN

Plastic Surgery of the Breast

What is plastic surgery of the breast?

What is the difference between silicone
and saline-filled implants?

What is breast reconstruction?

What are the health risks of this type
of plastic surgery?

More . . .

One of the most defining features of a woman's body is her breasts. Even when clothed, the appearance or prominence of breasts distinguish a man from a woman and greatly define a woman's figure. The subject of a woman's breasts is highly intimate, yet surgery of the breast is among the most debated of plastic surgery procedures. If you are considering plastic surgery of the breast, a public forum is not the place to get candid information specific to your goals. Consulting with a board-certified plastic surgeon experienced in breast surgery is where you should begin to gain information and answers to your questions.

Plastic surgery of the breast can alter the shape, size, and appearance of your breasts. It can also restore a more normal appearance to a breast that is deformed by surgery. It can improve breasts that are disproportionate to your body or to one another. Plastic surgery of the breast requires a woman to invest physically, emotionally, and financially in changing the appearance of her breasts. It can be unquestionably fulfilling for women who have the right motivations, realistic expectations and seek outcomes not for the moment, but for a lifetime.

40. What is plastic surgery of the breast?

Plastic surgery of the breast, much like any plastic surgery procedure, can be reconstructive (to restore a more normal appearance) or aesthetic (to enhance appearance).

Qualified providers

Plastic surgeons certified by the American Board of Plastic Surgery are the only qualified providers of plastic surgery of the breast. No other specialty has dedicated training specifically in plastic surgery procedures of the breast.

In choosing a plastic surgeon to perform any category of breast surgery, consider someone who is more than appropriately credentialed and skilled. Your plastic surgeon must be sensitive to your needs. He or she must also be very candid about your options and be realistic when defining the potential outcomes. All forms of plastic surgery have the potential for risks, complications, and sequelae. Breast surgery is no exception. The strength of a woman's desire to undergo breast surgery should be strong and sincere. Likewise, her surgeon's evaluation of her anatomy and her goals must be candid and thorough.

Categories and procedures

Aesthetic breast procedures include:

- Breast lift to reshape and reposition flattened breasts that hang low
- Breast augmentation to increase or enhance the size of breasts
- Breast reduction to reduce breast size for improved appearance only

Reconstructive breast procedures include:

- Post-mastectomy reconstruction to rebuild or restore a breast that has been surgically removed or disfigured by complete or partial mastectomy
- Breast reduction to reduce the size of overly large breasts, in disproportion to a woman's body, causing pain and discomfort

Following breast reconstruction, you are entitled to coverage for a procedure on the opposite breast to achieve symmetry between the breasts.

These are the most common breast procedures. There are additional, less common procedures that may be performed along with any of the above procedures or alone. These include correction of inverted nipples, nipple reduction, or reconstruction of breast anomalies such as correction of more than one nipple present on a single breast. In addition, congenital severe breast disproportion or asymmetry (caused by heredity, not by mastectomy) may be corrected through plastic surgery of the breast.

Your satisfaction

Patient studies show that women with very conservative enhancement of breast size or those with correction of even minor deformities are greatly satisfied with the results and feel immensely fulfilled. You don't need to undergo dramatic change to feel satisfied and fulfilled, and how you feel following any breast procedure can last a lifetime.

The outcomes of breast surgery may change over time as your body ages and weight fluctuates, however. Most importantly, any procedure that includes the use of a breast implant will need to be repeated over the course of a woman's lifetime, as breast implants are not considered permanent devices.

41. How can my breasts be enlarged?

Breast augmentation, also called augmentation mammaplasty, is surgery to enhance breast size through the placement of breast implants. Contrary to what we are led to believe by media and some celebrities who exploit their unnaturally excessive augmentation, most breast augmentation candidates don't desire overly large breasts. Most women seeking breast augmentation simply wish to bring proportion to the female body, to enhance a naturally small breast, or to restore breast volume loss due to pregnancy and/or breastfeeding.

Women who undergo breast augmentation by credentialed, skilled, experienced plastic surgeons report very high satisfaction, not only in appearance, but also in the way their breasts feel. Much of the key to your success in breast augmentation, as with any plastic surgery procedure, is to consult with a qualified, board-certified plastic surgeon. He or she should have experience in breast augmentation and other breast procedures. In addition, the surgeon you choose should listen carefully to your goals for surgery—the physical change you want to achieve and how you expect breast augmentation to enhance your quality of life.

Are you covered?

Breast augmentation is an aesthetic procedure. The only considerations for insurance coverage are to achieve symmetry when the opposite breast has been reconstructed after surgery to remove all or a portion of the breast (mastectomy).

Good candidates

Women of any age who are in good physical and emotional health are good candidates for breast augmentation. It should not, however, be performed in patients younger than 18 unless severe asymmetry exists.

Again, if the breast are severely sagging (ptotic), augmentation should not be performed without some form of breast lift (mastopexy).

Breast implants are not considered by the U.S. FDA to be lifetime devices. Realistic expectations for breast augmentation include accepting that during your lifetime your implants will need to be replaced.

How it's done

Breast implant size and shape is determined by a number of factors, namely the amount of increase in breast size you desire and how much breast tissue you naturally have. Also, the size of your frame and elasticity of your tissues may limit the size of implant that can be placed. Breast implants are measured in size by cubic

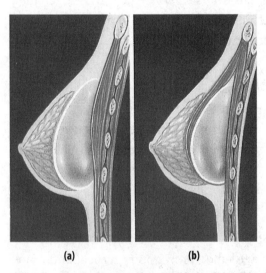

(a)   (b)

Figure 2   Breast augmentation. (a) subglandular; (b) submuscular. This is an artist's rendering and does not represent actual patient results. Individual results may vary. Courtesy of the American Society of Plastic Surgeons®. All rights reserved. Learn more at *www.plasticsurgery.org*.

centimeters (ccs) and can be pre-filled or may be filled once they are placed. Placement is either:

- Subglandular: above the chest muscle and below the breast tissue or glands
- Submuscular: below the chest muscle immediately on top of the chest wall

The location of the incisions through which implants are inserted depends on you and your plastic surgeon's preferences.

The most natural result occurs with submuscular placement. In addition, submuscular placement has a significantly lower rate of complication and a lower incidence of a condition called capsular contracture (a firm, irregular scar tissue that forms around the implant). Submuscular implant placement has a slightly longer recovery (2–3 more days) and may incur a bit more immediate post-operative discomfort. It also interferes less with mammogram readings than subglandular placement and is therefore considered more desireable for the long term. Subglandular placement, even of contoured implants, can result in a high curve at the top of the breast. This can make it obvious that a woman has breast implants, particularly when there is a significant increase in breast size.

The other option to consider is a choice of saline-filled or silicone gel implants. Question 42 specifically discusses the differences, advantages, and disadvantages to saline-filled and silicone gel implants.

The placement of implants and type of implants appropriate for you require that you carefully evaluate and discuss all of your options with your plastic surgeon.

Plastic Surgery of the Breast

What to expect

Breast augmentation is most commonly an outpatient procedure performed either under general anesthesia or local anesthesia with sedation, in an office-based, free-standing, ambulatory- or hospital-based surgical facility. An overnight hospital stay may be recommended in some cases.

When you awaken from surgery you will likely be stiff and sore. Tissues will be stretching to accommodate the breast implant and the swelling that occurs from the surgery itself. Most discomfort may be controlled with oral medications. Placement of a pain pump, which delivers medication directly to the surgical site may be recommended to control discomfort during the first 3 days after surgery. In some cases, small thin tubes may be placed at the incision sites to drain any excess fluid that might accumulate. You will be wearing a support bra, elastic bandage, or chest band for the first week or more following surgery, as recommended by your surgeon.

What you need to know

The risks and complications of breast augmentation include hematoma or blood pooling beneath the skin, breast tenderness, and heightened or lack of nipple sensation. A condition called capsular contracture that results in irregular and firm tissue surrounding the implant can also develop. There is a slight chance you may have unexpected milk production following insertion of implants. This may stop on its own or require medication. There is also the possibility of poorly healed or wide scars. Implants can be displaced, leak, or rupture. If they become infected, they must be removed. There are also the risks associated with anesthesia.

Early, mild cases of capsular contracture can be reduced with breast massage and/or minimal surgical release. In some cases it may be so severe that the scar tissue needs to be removed and the implant replaced. It can, however, reoccur. Capsular contracture may sometimes be the result of previous bleeding or a low-grade infection.

Leaking silicone gel implants may not readily be detected by decreased breast size but rather by hard knots in the breast, uneven appearance of the breasts, swelling, tenderness, numbness, or burning. If your implants are silicone, leaking implants may be diagnosed by magnetic resonance imaging (MRI) and should be removed even if the silicone is contained. Saline-filled implants simply deflate and are therefore easy to recognize and replace if treated early.

Your responsibilities

Prior to breast augmentation, patients over 30 years of age should have a baseline mammogram. Smokers should refrain from smoking for several weeks before surgery and during recovery. In addition, wearing your support bra as directed is imperative to proper healing. Even when your surgeon allows you to discontinue wearing a support bra, you may find wearing light support, such as a shelf bra or camisole, to be comfortable for sleeping.

Proper wound care and subsequent breast massage, as instructed by your plastic surgeon, may help to avoid capsular contracture and unsightly scars. Once healing is completed, an annual examination with your plastic surgeon to assess the condition of your implants and your breasts is also important. You should also have an annual exam with your gynecologist to check for breast changes and masses.

Your goals

The results of breast augmentation are visible immediately, although you will be somewhat swollen and your implants may temporarily appear higher than you might wish your final outcome to be. It may take a few months before implants settle to a final position. Breast augmentation should not interfere with a woman's ability to breast-feed, nor should it significantly alter the sensations in a woman's nipples. However, any surgery of the breast and more commonly, procedures with a periarealar incision (one around the dark skin surrounding the nipple) may result in these conditions.

Breast implants are not lifetime devices and, due to leaking or a change in breast tissue or aging, they will likely need to be replaced during a woman's lifetime. If a woman chooses to have implants removed and not replaced, the appearance of the breast will likely be changed, and sagging will occur just as it would after significant weight loss.

Diagnostic testing for breast health requires that you always let any health care professional know that you have implants. Implants may make mammograms more difficult to read. Different techniques must be used to displace the implant during a mammogram. This allows for a better image of the breast tissue and can help to avoid rupture of the implant from the breast compression necessary for mammography.

Your enhancement

Breast augmentation with implants has the advantage of slowing the natural aging or sagging process of the breasts in some women. However, where implant size is excessive, sagging and aging of the breasts can actually be exaggerated. Some women find they need not wear a bra and find new freedom and satisfaction in the way clothing fits and in new clothing options to enhance their figures.

There is no proven alternative to the placement of implants that enhances breast volume. Removing one's own fat from other areas of the body and injecting or implanting it to enlarge the breasts is a dangerous procedure that should not be performed. Marketed devices and herbal supplements to enhance breast size have not been proven to achieve permanent breast enhancement. The marketers of herbal supplements to enhance breast size are not subject to FDA approval or marketing regulations, and therefore their claims are unproven.

> Breast augmentation is the most commonly performed aesthetic plastic surgery procedure for women in the United States, as reported by the American Society of Plastic Surgeons, with over 254,000 procedures performed in 2003, a 20% increase since 2000.

> In 2003, ASPS reports that 45,147 breast implants for augmentation purposes only were removed, of which 81% were replaced. The most common cause of implant removal is, first, a patient's desire for a change in breast size, and second, implant rupture or leakage.

42. What is the difference between silicone gel and saline-filled breast implants?

There are many types of implants currently available to women. All have a solid silicone rubber-like outer shell that may be smooth or textured. Some may be rounded, and others may be contoured or sloped more like a natural breast. While there is debate among whether smooth or textured, rounded or contoured implants are your best choice, the greatest debate is between silicone gel and saline-filled implants.

Silicone gel implants, as of the writing of this book, are only used in the United States in breast reconstruction cases, in specific research studies, or to replace existing silicone implants. In October 2003, a U.S. FDA advisory panel recommended reinstatement of silicone breast implants as an option to any women seeking breast augmentation. The FDA, however, has chosen to wait for more long-term clinical studies to be completed and analyzed. The new generation of silicone implants currently under FDA review differ from those of the past in that they are filled with "cohesive" silicone—the silicone filler substance is not fluid, but instead it binds onto itself. Therefore, should the implants rupture or leak, there is less chance of free silicone in the body or the formation of granulomas. However, different manufacturers of silicone implant filler have different degrees of cohesion, and it is important that you ask specifically about the filler of any implant recommended for you. Although silicone breast implants have a more natural appearance and feel than saline breast implants, there is a higher rate of capsular contracture with hardness and deformity than with saline. Also, if silicone gel implants rupture and create pain or deformity, they should be surgically removed. Any free silicone should also be removed as much as possible to avoid hard nodules called granulomas. The procedure can be very involved and results in a significant recovery time.

On the other hand, when saline implants rupture, the saline is safely absorbed into a woman's body, and removal and replacement would be a relatively minor surgical procedure when treated early. The drawbacks of saline implants are that they are more defined and palpable, and they all wrinkle, even when over-filled. Wrinkling may be visible, particularly where breast tissue provides little coverage. The implants are generally not visible with clothing and rarely noticeable to other individuals. It is a myth that saline breast implants can make a sloshing noise as a woman moves her body.

Your choice in implants is best determined by discussing your options with your surgeon; new implant styles may be introduced by the implant manufacturers and approved by the U.S. FDA. Considerations include your lifestyle, the amount of enhancement you desire, and your personal preferences. Always request the package insert from your implants from your plastic surgeon, and make certain that you obtain and keep in a safe place the manufacturer's device sticker that identifies the brand of implant you received, its size, and the manufacturer's lot number and warranty.

In 1996, the Trilucent™ implant, filled with purified soybean oil, was introduced. In the United States about 200 women received this implant in an FDA-approved, controlled-research study. The study was ended in 1997 due to complications associated with the implant. No future plans for the implant exist.

According to data published by the U.S. Food & Drug Administration Center for Devices and Radiological Health, the following is reported with regard to health, implants with palpability (those that are more easily felt) are reported to be: textured implants, larger implants, subglandularly placed implants (on top of the chest muscle, below the breast glands), and implants in patients with smaller amounts of breast tissue. Also reported is that there is no greater risk of capsular contracture with a textured implants shell versus smooth implants.

43. Why were silicone gel breast implants recalled, and how do I determine whether any breast implants are right for me?

In the early 1990s, silicone gel breast implants were suspended from the market by the U.S. Food and Drug Administration (FDA) for first-time breast augmentation patients only. At issue was the theory that these implants contributed to connective tissue or autoimmune diseases (CTD) in some women (such as rheumatoid arthritis, lupus, and chronic fatigue syndrome). The FDA action was specific to the use of silicone gel implants in breast augmentation only. Some implant manufacturers voluntarily took their silicone gel implants off the market, pending safety review. However, some silicone gel implants have remained an available option for some breast reconstruction patients with specific procedural protocols, and for patients in formal research studies.

The U.S. FDA Breast Implants Information Update 2000 findings are reported on studies of silicone gel breast implants and possible links to illness in some women (*www.fda.gov.cdrh/breastimplants*). With regard to women having silicone gel implants and having signs and symptoms of CTDs, the report states, "It is unclear at this time whether the signs and symptoms experienced by these women are related to their implants." In addition, the findings of several independent studies are also reported, including one of the most comprehensive performed by researchers at Harvard Medical School in 1996. This study reported "a small but statistically insignificant risk of all CTDs reported by women with breast implants ... over a 10-year period, women with breast implants were 1.24 times more likely to report having a CTD or related disorder." The FDA further states, of all reported studies they reviewed, "When considered together, these studies indicate that the risk of developing a typical or defined CTD or related disorder due to having breast implants is low."

In 2003, an FDA advisory panel reviewed a petition from breast implant manufacturer Inamed Corporation to market a newer silicone gel implant. In October 2003, the panel voted that the FDA should approve, with conditions, their implant for use in breast reconstruction, breast augmentation, and revisional breast surgery procedures. In January of 2004, the FDA denied approval pending further information from Inamed.

Making your choice

It is your right to have breast implants, just as it is your right to accept any form of medical treatment. Research and the media should not influence your decision; they merely provide you with information. But the information does not come with instructions. Below are some guidelines for using this information and for making a decision that is right for you.

Your desire to have breast implants must be for your own personal fulfillment, not that of anyone else. Use media as a source for questions, not answers. Review the results of research published by unbiased patient advocate groups, such as the U.S. FDA, the National Institutes of Health, and recognized medical specialty societies such as the American Society of Plastic Surgeons.

Visit the Web sites of breast implant manufacturers or ask your plastic surgeon for specific data on the breast implants you are considering, published by that breast implant manufacturer. All public information published or advertised by a pharmaceutical company or a medical device manufacturer is subject to FDA review. These companies can be fined or have their products pulled from the market if they release false or biased information.

Now, take all your research and all your questions and have a discussion with a qualified, board-certified plastic surgeon with whom you feel comfortable and confident. Also, have a conversation with your personal physician if you wish. Gynecologists see only female patients, including those with breast implants. Talk to your doctor if you feel you need to. And talk to other women with breast implants. If you don't know a woman who has had breast implants, ask your surgeon or gynecologist for references to patients who do have implants, and talk to these women.

If you truly have the desire for breast augmentation or reconstruction using implants, make no decision until you go through the process of informed consent with your plastic surgeon. The process of informed consent is fully discussed in Question 20. It is your right to choose to have breast implants. Make certain your decision is purely your own.

The U.S. Food and Drug Administration established MedWatch to report "adverse events" thought to be associated with medical devices or drugs. With regard to silicone gel breast implants, if you experience a serious adverse effect that you and your physician believe is related to your breast implant, your surgeon should complete a MedWatch form 3500, provide you with a copy, and submit this to the FDA. Medwatch forms are available at *http://www.fda.gov/medwatch/index.html*.

44. What can be done to restore breast shape and position?

Heredity and aging can cause a woman's breasts to sag or flatten. But ptosis (sagging of the breast) is more often the result of a reduction in breast volume, either from weight loss or the breast changes associated with pregnancy and breastfeeding. In higher degrees of ptosis, the nipple and areola of the breast hang lower than the breast crease. For women who are considering breast lift surgery or "mastopexy," a support bra is necessary to keep the breasts in a more normal position. They want their breasts to be more "perky" so that they no longer have to wear a bra with all their clothing or wear bathing suits with support.

Breast lift changes the breast to a more youthful shape and position. It repositions the nipple to a higher location, with a more natural point of projection. Also, it can reduce the size of the areola (the darker skin surrounding the nipple). Breast lift does not normally change the volume of breasts, only breast shape and position. In some cases a very small reduction of breast volume may be performed on one or both breasts. In other cases, a breast implant may be placed for enlargement and to achieve a firmer breast.

Are you covered?

Breast lift is a purely aesthetic procedure and is generally not eligible for insurance coverage. Coverage is possible only when it is performed to achieve symmetry when the other breast is reconstructed following mastectomy or other breast cancer surgery.

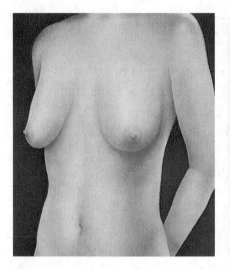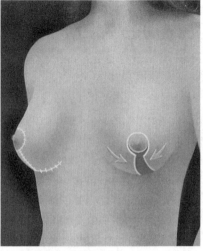

Figure 3   Breast Lift (mastopexy). This is an artist's rendering and does not represent actual patient results. Individual results may vary. Courtesy of the American Society of Plastic Surgeons®. All rights reserved. Learn more at *www.plasticsurgery.org*.

Good candidates

Any woman who desires to improve the shape and position of her breasts, who is in general good health, and who has realistic expectations for the outcomes of surgery is a good a candidate for breast lift. Women who may have future pregnancies might consider postponing a breast lift. While breast lift may not affect breast-feeding, the results of your surgery can be significantly diminished by the changes in the breasts that occur during pregnancy and breast-feeding.

How it's done

Breast lift requires incisions on the breast to reduce excess skin of the breast and areola and to reshape the deep tissues of the breast. It restores firmness and raises the breast and nipple to a higher, more natural position. Your incision pattern will be based on the amount of correction that will achieve your goals, the quality of your skin tone, the size of the areola, and the location of the nipple. If a reduction in the size of your areola is necessary, you will require an incision around the perimeter of the areola. A full examination and candid discussion with your plastic surgeon is the best strategy for defining an incision pattern that is right for you.

Once the incisions are made, the underlying breast tissue will be reshaped and deep sutures may be used to hold the breast tissue in place. The areola is reduced in circumference when appropriate. Excess skin is removed and the nipple, which remains attached, is raised to a higher position. The skin is brought together and sutured to achieve your new breast shape and position. Removable or dissolving sutures may be used to close the incisions.

What to expect

Beast lift most likely will be performed with general anesthesia or local anesthesia with sedation. Local anesthesia may be used in some cases where a small elevation of the nipple is required. The procedure will be performed in an office-based, freestanding ambulatory or hospital-based surgical facility and is routinely done on an outpatient basis.

You may awaken from surgery wearing a support bra or elastic bandage that you will continue to wear as recommended by your plastic surgeon. Small tubes may be placed at the incision sites to allow any excess fluid accumulation to drain; these will likely be in place for 1 to 2 days. You will be sore and experience discomfort at the incision sites following surgery. However, this discomfort can easily be controlled with medication.

You may resume light normal activity as soon as you feel ready and should be walking the day of surgery. But you will want to avoid lifting anything heavy or making any jerking or pulling motions for the first few days following surgery. If you have nonabsorbable sutures, they will be removed in a week or two following surgery. You may be given silicone tapes or gel to apply to your scars to reduce the formation of raised, red, firm, or other undesirable scars.

What you need to know

The risks of breast lift include the development of thick or wide scars. Blood pooling beneath the skin (called a hematoma) that may need to be drained is possible. A loss of nipple sensation or temporary sensitivity is possible. In addition, there is the risk of infection; however, this is rare. As with any surgical procedure, there are risks associated with anesthesia.

Your responsibilities

Smoking can significantly affect your ability to heal, and any patient who smokes should stop smoking for several weeks before surgery and during recovery. Following all instructions for wound cleansing, massage of scars and the use of tapes or topical ointments can improve the appearance of scars and lessen the chance of forming raised or firm scars. Following all instructions for wearing support garments is essential to your breasts to heal properly. Some women wear a support camisole when sleeping and if this is comfortable for you, it can only enhance and help to maintain the results of your breast lift.

Your goals

The results of breast lift surgery are visible immediately, although breast shape will continue to settle for several months. Final results, including the softening and fading of scars, may take as much as 1 to 2 years. Scars will always be visible; however, they are usually hidden under most swimsuits and bras.

Breast lift should not interfere with your ability to breastfeed and will rarely alter normal breast sensations. Breast lift surgery is not completely permanent; breasts may sag or lose elasticity over time as the result of natural aging. You can help to maintain your results by maintaining a stable weight.

Proven lift

Women who undergo breast lift find new confidence not only in their appearance when clothed, but also without clothing. Despite the visible scars on the breast, the more youthful and shapely appearance of the breast can be very fulfilling and appealing.

If you want greater breast volume in addition to improved breast shape and position, breast augmentation can be performed along with breast lift. The placement of implants is the only way of increasing breast size, but implants are not an alternative to breast lift. In fact, there is no alternative to breast lift. Placement of implants alone may somewhat alter breast shape and

Breast lift is the least common of breast procedures. The American Society of Plastic Surgeons reported nearly 67,000 procedures performed in 2003.

improve firmness; however, low breast or nipple position can only be corrected through breast lift. No topical firming creams, exercise, or devices have been proven to improve, raise, or restore breast shape.

45. What can be done to make my breasts smaller?

Breast reduction is surgery performed to reduce the size of large breasts, bring the nipples to a more natural position, and make the areola (the pigmented area around the nipple) a more normal size. The goals of breast reduction are not only to improve proportion in the female figure, but also to alleviate associated physical symptoms. These symptoms include:

- Back, neck, and shoulder pain
- Deep painful grooves that develop in the shoulders from the bras required for support
- Rashes and skin irritation that can develop under the breast creases
- Pain in the breast itself as the weight of pendulous breast tissue pulls the breast downward

Breast reduction, technically called reduction mammaplasty, can be an immensely fulfilling procedure. In most cases, breast reduction can free a woman of the pain and restricted physical activities associated with large, pendulous breasts. To better understand a woman's desire for and the fulfillment and outcomes of breast reduction surgery, the American Society of Plastic Surgeons has posted findings by the Breast Reduction Assessment and Value of Outcomes study (BRAVO) conducted by the Plastic Surgery Educational Foundation (on its Web site, *www.plasticsurgery.org*). The Web site also includes patient experiences and first-hand accounts of how breast reduction surgery has enhanced the quality of life for some women.

Not only does breast reduction improve the proportion of a woman's body but, as a result, your posture may also improve. And the freedom from excess breast weight and size will allow you to wear many different styles of clothing that you previously could not wear. In addition, you might find an increased desire for fitness, ability to participate in sports, and even the confidence to wear a swimsuit.

Are you covered?

Breast reduction is often considered a reconstructive procedure. However, insurance coverage of any procedure must be precertified, and coverage varies among insurance companies. Most commonly, the standards for reimbursement or insurance coverage of breast reduction are defined by the insurer based on the volume of breast tissue to be removed and other criteria (such as height, weight, previous medical treatment for pain, etc.). Some insurers may deny coverage altogether.

Debate and lobbying for a uniform standard among insurers for coverage of breast reduction has been an ongoing effort of the American Society of Plastic Surgeons. However, the most appropriate standard would have to take into account the proportion of breast size to a woman's body. For example, a very small-framed woman with large breasts may suffer greatly from breasts that may only need to be reduced by 500 grams. Other women may have far in excess of 1000

Plastic Surgery of the Breast

grams removed to achieve their goals. Only examination by and discussion of your goals with a qualified plastic surgeon will determine just what degree of breast reduction is appropriate for you and, ultimately, it is your insurer that determines whether or not your procedure qualifies for reimbursement.

Good candidates

Good candidates for breast reduction surgery are women with no serious health problems, who are of relatively normal weight despite their overly large breasts, and whose breast development has generally reached maturity (usually around age 18). The reason for waiting until breast development is nearly completed is that additional breast growth may significantly change the outcomes of breast reduction surgery. Breast reduction can be performed at an earlier age, but your results may likely change and you may need additional surgery in the future.

Likewise, women who are planning to have children in the near future might consider delaying breast reduction, as pregnancy and nursing can result in changes of the breast. Significant weight gain and loss, plus various hormones, can also affect breast size and the need for additional procedures.

Women of any age can be candidates for breast reduction surgery, as long as they accept that over time the outcomes of surgery can change somewhat. Any candidate for breast reduction should accept that along with the benefits come permanent scars. There is also the possible loss of nipple sensation or inability to breast-feed.

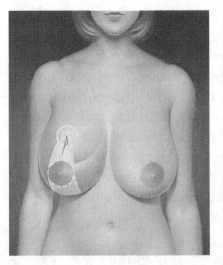
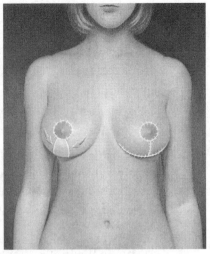

Figure 4   Breast Reduction (reduction mammaplasty) This is an artist's rendering and does not represent actual patient results. Individual results may vary. Courtesy of the American Society of Plastic Surgeons®. All rights reserved. Learn more at *www.plasticsurgery.org*.

How it's done

Breast reduction can be performed using one of three procedural techniques:

- Surgical excision with pedicle techniques, where the nipple's blood vessels and nerves stay attached while the other tissue is excised.
- Liposuction techniques to reduce excess breast fat only (not glandular tissue), performed alone or in conjunction with surgical excision of breast tissue and skin.
- Surgical excisions and nipple grafting which removes the nipple and excess tissues, then grafts the nipple into position on the newly formed breast; this procedure is rarely necessary.

Where breast reduction is more limited, and not likely to classify for insurance reimbursement, liposuction techniques alone may reduce breast size by removing excess fat deposits in and around the breast. While liposuction may reduce breast size, it does not reduce excess skin, nor does it change nipple position or reduce areolar size. This may be an important part or your breast reduction goals. Therefore, if it is recommended that you have breast reduction by liposuction techniques alone, you should know what can and cannot be achieved. You should have skin with good elasticity and breasts that, while large, are not pendulous or stretched downward.

Where breasts are not only disproportionately large but also stretch downward, excision of breast tissue, fat, and skin is the more appropriate breast reduction procedure. Excisional procedures will reduce the breast size, improve the breast shape, reduce the areola, and raise the breast and nipple position. Except in very rare circumstances, a "pedicle" technique should always be used. Pedicle means the blood and nerve supply to the nipple are maintained rather than detached. As a result, the nipple continues to have sensation and erection.

The alternative to pedicle techniques is nipple grafting. With this technique, the areola and nipple are removed, the breast volume is reduced by excising tissue and the nipple is then attached in a different location. Breast reduction in this manner is for very pendulous breasts where a pedicle may not be possible to achieve desired breast shape or nipple position. It is also appropriate when nipple viability (the ability of the nipple to survive) is questionable during a pedicle procedure. With nipple grafting, there will no longer be any erotic sensation or erection of the nipple. It is, therefore, never the procedure of choice in someone who is a good candidate for a pedicle procedure.

Determining the amount of tissue to reduce requires candid conversation with your plastic surgeon. Your goals for size, proportion, and comfort should be discussed along with the amount of tissue removal necessary for insurance coverage. Breast reduction can result in dramatic change in breast size, from a DD cup to as small as an A cup. However, most women want to have a B or C cup postoperatively.

Note that breast reduction may not be necessary on both breasts. Where severe asymmetry exists in the breasts, only one breast may require reduction to match the size of the other. But unless a mastopexy (breast lift) or other procedure is performed on the opposite breast, the shape of the breasts and nipple position may not be symmetrical.

What to expect

Breast reduction will likely be performed under general anesthesia, and depending on the extent of your reduction, may include an overnight hospital stay. You will awaken from surgery wearing a support bra or elastic support bandages, and small thin drainage tubes may be placed near the incision sites to drain any fluid and blood that accumulates during the first few days following surgery. You will experience discomfort at the incision sites. You may also find that the back, neck, and shoulder pain you had before surgery is greatly relieved. Surgical discomfort can usually be controlled with oral medications. You will be encouraged to begin walking as soon as possible following surgery, although your physical activity will be restricted for several days as healing continues. You will be advised not to lift anything heavy or do anything that results in a jerking or pulling motion. When sleeping, it is recommended you lie in an elevated position.

You may be required to wear a support bra or elastic bandages around the clock for a few weeks following surgery to support your breasts as they heal. Drains may be removed within 1 to 3 days following surgery. Stitches will be removed no longer than 2 weeks following surgery.

Within 2 weeks following surgery or as soon as you feel ready, you can return to normal activity, as long as you don't engage in heavy lifting, running, or anything that may cause bouncing or trauma to the breast as it continues to heal.

What you need to know

It is important to know that bleeding, blood clots, loss of sensation in the nipples, or infection can occur. Poorly healed or thick scars may develop and may need to be surgically corrected. In very rare cases, the nipple may be lost, requiring later reconstruction.

Your obligations

Smokers are at greater risk for poor healing of incisions and will be required to stop smoking for several weeks before surgery and throughout the recovery process. Following your plastic surgeon's instructions for wound care, wearing required garments, and following prescribed activity restrictions is essential for a good outcome. You may be advised to use silicone tapes, massage, and/or topical treatments to reduce the chance of raised red scars.

Even when your surgeon allows you to discontinue use of a support bra during the night, wearing a camisole with built-in support or a "shelf" bra at night can improve your comfort and decrease tension on the breast wounds. And while clothing options are greatly limited following breast reduction, to include such things as halters, it is a good idea to include some form of breast support with any garment you wear.

Your goals

The results of breast reduction surgery are visible immediately following surgery, although it may take several months for all the swelling to diminish. It will take up to a year for breast position to fully settle, and it may take up to two years for scars to fade. However, know that scars will always be visible after surgery.

Breast reduction, when performed using pedicle techniques, will likely not interfere with a woman's ability to breast-feed, although this is not always assured. While it is less likely for a woman to lose breast sensation with pedicle techniques, it is still possible to have reduced or impaired breast sensation and nipple function.

Your freedom

Many women are amazed at how significantly breast reduction can improve their quality of life, allowing them to live free of daily pain and discomfort. They can engage in physical activities that were once impossible due to the size and weight of their breasts. You may not only find yourself shopping for new bras, but also new clothing in styles that you previously would have never considered buying.

According to the American Society of Plastic Surgeons, in 2003 breast reduction was 5th among most-common reconstructive plastic surgery procedures performed, with just over 113,000 procedures. That was a steady increase of 10,000 or more procedures over the preceding three years. The American Society for Aesthetic Plastic Surgery reported 125,600 procedures in that same year—the discrepancy is likely due to the fact that breast reduction was counted in both reconstructive and cosmetic cases.

46. Can I improve a breast disfigured by or lost due to breast cancer surgery?

Breast reconstruction is surgery to restore or rebuild a breast that is either disfigured or completely removed due to disease, including breast cancer and some benign breast disorders. Any woman facing lumpectomy or total mastectomy should evaluate the possibility of breast reconstruction prior to her undergoing the ablative surgery. In most cases, mastectomy or tumor removal is performed by a cancer surgeon or general surgeon. If a plastic surgeon is consulted prior to surgery, the best strategic plan for reconstruction can be determined. It may be best to begin reconstruction at the time of mastectomy or at a later date, depending on your health and your surgeon's preferences.

Techniques for breast reconstruction

Reconstruction, or rebuilding the breast mound, can be achieved through one of four techniques:

- Use of a breast implant, often in conjunction with a technique called tissue expansion

- A latissimus dorsi flap, using a woman's own muscle, fat, and skin from her back, often in conjunction with an implant
- A TRAM, or transverse rectus abdominus musculocutaneous flap, using a woman's own muscle, fat, and skin from her abdomen
- A free flap, using a woman's own muscle, fat, and skin from the buttocks, abdomen, or thigh, transplanted to the chest wall using microsurgical techniques

All of these procedures result in creation of the breast mound, often through more than one stage. Creation of a nipple requires an additional procedure, typically through grafting and/or tattooing techniques. Determining what procedure is right for you is highly individualized based on your degree of deformity, the condition of any remaining breast tissue, your physical build, and your health. All of these factors will be considered for your plastic surgeon to make a recommendation for reconstruction. Your plastic surgeon will also take into consideration your personal preference and goals for reconstruction; however, realize that not all procedures for reconstruction are appropriate options in every case. Also, your plastic surgeon may feel more comfortable with the results he or she can obtain with some procedures and not others. Very few plastic surgeons, for instance, do free flaps for breast reconstruction.

Are you covered?

Most women do not know, and often are not told, that insurance companies are required by law to cover *any* procedures of breast reconstruction if they cover the ablative surgery (partial or full mastectomy). This includes procedures determined by your plastic surgeon to achieve symmetry between the breasts following breast cancer surgery. The enactment of this law is directly a result of the patient advocacy efforts led by the American Society of Plastic Surgeons that not only mandated coverage for breast reconstruction, but also for additional procedures on the opposite breast necessary for achieving symmetry. Today any woman who undergoes mastectomy is entitled to coverage for reconstruction by her insurer. Precertification may be required, and your surgeon's office will provide the documentation necessary for coverage or assist you in filing for insurance coverage.

> The exact text of the 1998 Federal Breast Reconstruction Law and any updates to the law can be accessed at *http://www.plastic surgery.org/public_education/Breast-Reconstruction-Resources-1998-Federal-Law.cfm.*

> The American Society of Plastic Surgeons maintains a state-by-state update of laws related to breast reconstruction that can be found at: *http://www.plasticsurgery.org/public_education/Breast-Reconstruction-Resources-State-Laws.cfm.*

Good candidates and timing

Candidates for surgical breast reconstruction are determined by four factors:

- individual desire
- physician recommendations
- timing
- general health

The process of breast reconstruction can sometimes begin at the time of mastectomy or lumpectomy. Reconstruction may be delayed depending on your course of nonsurgical treatments (chemotherapy or radiation therapy) or based on the recommendation of your oncologist. It may also be delayed if that is your preference.

The ability to awaken from mastectomy with the beginnings of a new breast mound already in place can be immensely important to a woman and may greatly improve her road to health. Therefore, it is important to consider breast reconstruction before undergoing mastectomy. Discuss this with your breast surgeon, and, if feasible, consult with a plastic surgeon as soon as possible. Dealing with breast cancer or tumor removal is a very difficult process. But pursing the options available to make you whole again will allow you to return to your normal life more quickly. Your emotional and physical health will benefit greatly.

How it's done

Breast reconstruction begins with a careful evaluation of your condition and a discussion of options recommended by your plastic surgeon. The discussion will include whether you are a good candidate for reconstruction, the procedure that your plastic surgeon feels is right for you, and the timing of the procedure.

Most breast reconstruction procedures to create the breast mound will be performed under general anesthesia and will likely be in a hospital with a one night stay or more. Secondary procedures such as nipple grafting may be performed in your surgeon's office, an office-based or ambulatory surgical facility, or in a hospital as an outpatient procedure.

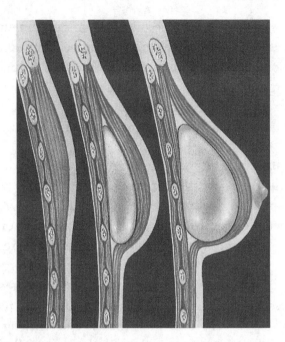

Figure 5   Breast reconstruction: Tissue expansion. This is an artist's render-ing and does not represent actual patient results. Individual results may vary. Courtesy of the American Society of Plastic Surgeons®. All rights reserved. Learn more at *www.plasticsurgery.org*.

Implant and expansion

The use of a breast implant to reconstruct the breast mound first requires enough healthy tissue to cover and support the implant, often achieved through tissue expansion.

Tissue expansion begins with placement of a medical-grade, silicone-shelled balloon that over time is filled with sterile saline solution through an internal, one-way valve. As the balloon is filled and increases in size, it creates new cells and stretches the overlying skin and other tissue. It may take as many as 6 months to achieve the final size, and discomfort will accompany the expansion process.

Once the process of tissue expansion is completed, the existing expander may be replaced with a final breast implant. Some types of expanders may also serve as the final implant.

What to expect

Initial placement of the expander will result in discomfort that can be controlled with oral medications or a pain pump. The discomfort should lessen significantly in the first 3 to 4 days following surgery. Sleeping or lying in an elevated position is recommended for your comfort. You should be ready for light, normal activity within 3 to 4 days following surgery. Stitches will usually be removed within 10 days following surgery. Your incision sites will be red, and may be raised and itchy for some time following surgery. Massage of the incision site and application of silicone sheeting or special scar-reducing topical ointments, such as Mederma®, may improve the condition of scars.

Once the expander is placed, you will have frequent visits to your plastic surgeon to gradually increase the amount of fluid in the expander. The process of filling the expander and stretching tissues can be uncomfortable; over-the-counter medications or prescription medications can make you more comfortable.

When the tissue expander is replaced with an implant, you may have similar sensation but less discomfort than the tissue expansion stage. Moreover, you can expect permanent, visible scars to remain on the breast mound. Plastic surgeons will attempt to place these scars so that they are concealed by a bathing suit or bra cup, but sometimes the location of the tumor that was removed does not permit this.

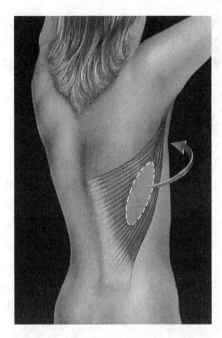

Figure 6   Latissimus dorsi flap. This is an artist's rendering and does not represent actual patient results. Individual results may vary. Courtesy of the American Society of Plastic Surgeons®. All rights reserved. Learn more at *www.plasticsurgery.org.*

Latissimus dorsi flap

When a woman does not have enough of her own breast tissue to support an implant, or if she has had radiation therapy or previous infections, tissue expansion may not be feasible. A latissimus dorsi flap may be a recommended alternative in these cases. The flap uses muscle and overlying tissue taken from a woman's own back that maintains its original blood and nerve supply. It is brought under the armpit, through a tunnel to a woman's chest. The flap is generally very hardy and can support a breast implant. In a few select cases it may provide enough tissue to create a breast mound without an implant.

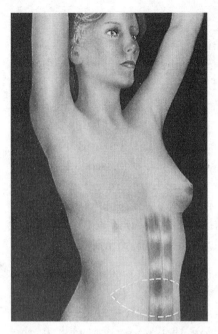 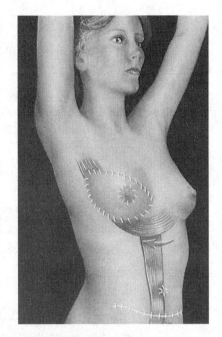

Figure 7 Tram flap procedure. This is an artist's rendering and does not represent actual patient results. Individual results may vary. Courtesy of the American Society of Plastic Surgeons®. All rights reserved. Learn more at *www.plasticsurgery.org*.

TRAM flap

A TRAM flap uses skin, muscle, and fat taken from a woman's abdomen that remains attached to the original blood and nerve supply. A TRAM flap may not be appropriate in cases where a woman has an excess of abdominal fat or previous abdominal surgeries. The flap is tunneled up to the breast mound site and provides enough tissue to create the completely reconstructed breast. Generally, a second stage is required for final shaping of the breast. A side benefit to a TRAM flap procedure is that the patient will gain a tummy tuck.

Free flaps

Where no other method of breast reconstruction is appropriate, some plastic surgeons will perform breast reconstruction using free flaps. Tissue can be completely detached from the buttocks, thigh, or abdomen, along with nerve and blood supplies, and transplanted to the breast mound site using microsurgical techniques to attach the blood vessels and nerves to those at the new site. Free flaps are generally used when other flaps will not result in adequate tissue to create a breast mound. Any free flap technique will most commonly create the full breast mound.

What you need to know

Infection and bleeding are among the complications of any breast reconstruction techniques, as well as the risks associated with anesthesia. In addition, flap techniques risk loss of tissue at either the reconstructed breast mound or the donor site. The use of implants includes the risk of a condition called capsular contracture, where excess scar tissue forms around the implant causing a very hard physical touch and unnatural appearance. In addition, the use of any breast implant carries the risk of implant leakage or rupture requiring the implant be removed and replaced if you wish. Any of these conditions may require further surgery. In addition, infection or exposure of an implant may require revision with a flap technique.

Your obligations

A woman undergoing breast reconstruction has many responsibilities regarding the reconstruction process. Smokers must stop smoking for several weeks before and throughout the reconstruction process. Continuing visits with your plastic surgeon and following all of your physician's instructions are imperative.

Your goals

The outcomes of breast reconstruction are immensely fulfilling. Plastic surgeons can make a breast appear very natural, but the feel of the breast to the physical touch and sensation will not mirror a natural breast. You will lack nipple sensation, if it has been removed during mastectomy, and the ability for a nipple erection. A woman who has undergone breast reconstruction will not be able to breastfeed from the reconstructed breast.

Scars will always remain on the breast site from the mastectomy and at the donor site if flaps are used.

Your health requires a long relationship with your oncologist. A continuing relationship with your plastic surgeon is also important, particularly in cases where implants are used for breast reconstruction.

Alternatives

There is no alternative to surgical reconstruction of the breast that allows a woman to have a breast that is part of the body. An external prosthesis is a non-surgical alternative held in place by an undergarment. It is not part of a woman's body. This type of prosthesis can be uncomfortable and prevent a woman from wearing certain kinds of clothing.

According the American Society of Plastic Surgeons, breast reconstruction procedures numbered nearly 69,000 in 2003. That is a slow and steady decline over recent years. The likely cause is an increase in the number of lumpectomies for small tumors and a decrease in the number of mastectomies.

According to a study reported by the American Cancer Society in November, 2000, led by researchers at the University of Michigan, "women who have breast reconstruction after a mastectomy report significant psychological and emotional benefits." Timing of breast reconstruction was reported to affect those benefits; however, the techniques used—with or without placement of a breast implant—did not appear to make much of a difference in a woman's level of satisfaction.

In 2003, ASPS reported that over 17,341 breast implants used in breast reconstruction were surgically removed, of which 73% were replaced.

The National Institutes of Health reports nearly 165,000 women were diagnosed with breast cancer in 2000. That same year, over 80,000 breast reconstruction procedures were performed. The assumption is that somewhat less than half of all women who are diagnosed with breast cancer will undergo reconstruction. However, of those diagnosed, there are missing data on the number of those with mastectomy versus lumpectomy [also called breast-conserving surgery].

At present there are no statistics that define how many women diagnosed with breast cancer received information about breast reconstruction. Some studies estimate that as many as one-third to one-half of women who undergo some form of surgery to remove a portion of or a complete breast due to disease do not receive any information about reconstruction.

47. Will plastic surgery of the breast increase my risk of breast disease?

There is no proven link between any form of breast surgery, including surgery with implants, and breast disease. The National Institutes of Health and National Cancer Institute as well as the U.S. Food & Drug Administration (FDA) at the time of publication of this book had no statement linking breast surgery to breast disease, nor data linking women who have undergone breast surgery of any type to breast disease. The U.S. Institutes of Medicine reported in 2000 that breast cancer is no more common in women with implants than those without implants. In addition, in April 2001 researchers at the National Cancer Institutes issued a report stating, "women with silicone breast implants were not at increased risk for most cancers." The study specifically stated that no increased risk was found for sarcoma, Hodgkin or non-Hodgkin lymphoma, or multiple myeloma.

With regard to illnesses other than breast cancer, the U.S. FDA Center for Devices and Radiological Health reported in 2000 that most studies of the illnesses women with breast implants report as believed to be linked to their implants, "have failed to show an association with breast implants." Further, there is no information that breast implants may be damaging to children born of mothers with implants (silicone gel or saline filled) who breastfed or did not. However, studies do suggest that breast implants can in some cases impede the ability of a woman to breast-feed. How often this occurs is not known. Additionally, research reported by the FDA in 1998 found that silicon levels in breast milk of women with silicone gel breast implants was the same when compared with breast milk from women without implants.

Capsular contracture is the only breast condition unquestionably linked to breast implants. Capsular contracture is not breast disease, however, but excess scar tissue that forms around the implant. The condition can occur with any type of implanted device in the body, and it can be minimized and corrected in nearly every case.

In fact, women who have had breast surgery of any kind are more likely to practice breast self-examination (BSE) and be more in tune with the feel and form of their breast tissue. Women who have undergone reconstruction will certainly have breast tissue that feels different from a natural breast. Women who have undergone breast reduction will have an easier time with BSE as there is less tissue to examine. Both breast reduction and breast lift patients will have a slight change in the feel of breast tissue. However, this does not complicate BSE or mammograms.

In a report by the Mayo clinic, women with saline breast implants found it easier to do breast self exam.

The implants separated breast tissue from the body, making changes in breast tissue more apparent.

Women with overly large breasts may, in fact, gain health benefits and reduce the risk of breast cancer, by undergoing breast reduction surgery.

Questions about any breast surgery procedure or breast implants and related topics of health can be found at *http://www.nlm.nih.gov/ medlineplus/breastimplantsbreastreconstruction.html,* the Medline medical library resource of the U.S. National Institutes of Health.

Plastic Surgery of the Breast

PART EIGHT

A Better Body: Surgical Body Contouring

What is body contouring?

What is liposuction, and how can it reduce fat?

What is a tummy tuck?

Can sagging skin be corrected with plastic surgery?

More ...

Most of us need to sweat a little (or a lot) to maintain a fit and attractive body. The results of heredity, aging, and significant weight loss can all immensely affect the physical contours of the body regardless of how much we exercise. For women, add pregnancy to the mix and the result may be disproportionate body contours caused by excess fat deposits, sagging or loose skin, and even separated muscles.

Female breast surgery clearly changes body contours. However, due to the specialized nature of the female breast, these procedures are in a category of their own. All other plastic surgery procedures that change the shape or appearance of the body fall into the category of "body contouring."

48. What is body contouring?

Body contouring is plastic surgery that reshapes or changes the physical appearance of the body. It includes procedures that generally:

• Remove excess fat from the body
• Reduce excess skin and other tissue from the body
• Enhance small body contours

Body contouring is designed to bring better proportion to the body. In some cases, body contouring procedures do more than improve the appearance of the body. For example, a tummy tuck can correct an abdominal muscle separation called diastasis. And while most of us wish to look slimmer and trimmer, there are some people who seek to augment body contours through implants that change and enhance the size of specific regions of the body.

Augmentation of body contours is more popular in European and Latin American countries, but is gaining interest in the United States. In 2003 "butt implants" were identified by WebMD as one of "7 New Trends in Cosmetic Surgery" (*www.webmd.com*).

Surgical body contouring

Body contouring is achieved through surgical techniques that accomplish one of the following:

- Removal of fat through suctioning (liposuction)
- Direct reduction of skin and/or fat
- Change of muscle position
- Enhancement using implants
- Enhancement using your own tissues

Body contouring is achieved through surgery. There are no proven nonsurgical means that can accomplish the same results as body contouring. Regular exercise will firm, tone, and increase muscles; diet and/or exercise can help you lose weight. The results of exercise and weight loss can reshape your body. But no amount of exercise or diet can correct sagging skin that results following major weight loss or that develops as we age. Nor can diet or exercise remove excess familial fat deposits, those that result from heredity and accumulate in certain areas of your body.

As you read this section on body contouring procedures, you may wonder why you cannot find reference to "innovative" and "one-of-a-kind" medical treatments that are advertised to improve the appearance of your body. Only recognized body contouring procedures taught in accredited residency, fellowship, and continuing medical education programs are discussed in this book. These include:

- Liposuction to remove fat, including the tumescent and ultrasound-assisted techniques
- Treatment of excess male breast tissue (gynecomastia)
- Tummy tuck, to improve the abdominal shape and change the position of or repair abdominal muscles
- Body lifts, to reduce excess skin, tissues, and fat of the body and reposition remaining tissues
- Brachioplasty to surgically reshape loose and drooping upper arm
- Augmentation, which uses implants or fat to increase the curves, contours, and size of the buttocks, calves, and thighs. (Breast augmentation is covered explicitly in Part 7: Breast Surgery.)
- Combinations of the above procedures to refine the appearance of the body, particularly following major weight loss

49. Is body contouring an alternative to weight loss and exercise?

Body contouring procedures may reduce the size of body contours, but they are *not* intended to be an alternative to losing weight. The only reason body contouring may result in some weight loss is that some body contouring procedures remove tissue (and thus weight) from the body.

Body contouring is not the solution to achieving a better body for people who are obese, in poor health, or who do not practice healthy eating habits and appropriate exercise. For body contouring to be safe and effective, you need to be in good physical condition. There is no point in reshaping your body if your weight is unstable and you are not committed to the practices that will keep your weight stable and your body reasonably fit. Moreover, if you are obese or in poor health, you are at risk for a difficult recovery and unsatisfactory outcome. And if your bad habits persist, any benefit you gain from body contouring surgery will be short-lived. Alternatively, maintaining a healthy and active lifestyle will result in long-term improvements, affected only by aging and weight changes (including pregnancy).

50. How can fat be reduced?

Liposuction, also called lipoplasty or suction lipectomy, is surgery that uses vacuum suction and special instruments to remove localized, subcutaneous fat deposits. Subcutaneous refers to the fat that exists immediately below the skin and above muscle. Familial fat deposits are those caused by heredity and that remain despite diet and exercise. Fit individuals with familial fat deposits are good candidates for liposuction. Liposuction also improves body contours in people who simply have disproportionate fat deposits in specific localized areas. These areas generally include:

- Fat in the neck that gives the appearance of a chin that disappears into the neck or a double chin
- A lower body that is out of proportion with the upper body
- Tummy, hips, thighs, buttocks knees, ankles, or upper arms that have disproportionate bulges and irregular contours

- Male breasts that appear almost woman-like, having excess curves

Liposuction may also be used as a technique in female breast reduction; the procedure and all appropriate techniques to reduce the size of the female breast are fully discussed in Question 45.

Liposuction removes excess fat and will reduce certain contours, but it does not reduce skin. Therefore, good candidates for liposuction have healthy, elastic skin that can contract to the newly formed contours following surgery. Where skin does not conform or shrink back to the new, smaller body contours, surgical techniques such as body lifts may be needed in conjunction with or following liposuction.

Liposuction cannot correct cellulite, a dimpled appearance on the skin of the buttocks, hips, and thighs of some women. In fact, in some cases, cellulite may become worse to a degree. Why? Because cellulite exists above the fat deposits that are suctioned. When these areas are suctioned or reduced, the loss of volume beneath the skin may cause the dimpled appearance of cellulite to be even more pronounced.

Liposuction was first developed in Europe in the 1980s as a procedure to surgically suction excess fat deposits from the body. It was primarily used in the hips, thighs, and buttocks. The cannula, or thin hollow surgical metal tube inserted under the skin to remove fat, was large (10 mm in diameter or more) and blunt-tipped. The cannula was vigorously thrust back and forth to loosen large areas of subcutaneous fat (fat immediately below the skin surface) and was attached to flexible tubing, connected to vacuum suction to achieve reduction of localized fat.

Liposuction still uses a cannula and suction to dislodge and remove fat from the body, but more refined techniques have been developed. For instance, with the advent of tumescence, smaller cannulas are used to remove a greater total volume of fat and to sculpt smoother contours. In recent years, new techniques such as ultrasound-assisted liposuction have been developed, which also allow for improved sculpting. Both of these techniques and their advantages and applications are discussed specifically in this chapter.

In some cases, liposuction may be performed using a syringe attached to the cannula to draw out subcutaneous fat. The collected fat may then be used to augment other areas of your body. This procedure is called autologous fat injection or fat transfer (discussed in Part 11).

Who performs liposuction?

You must fully understand the following before choosing a qualified provider for liposuction. There is no legislative means to control who performs liposuction in the United States. Furthermore, liposuction equipment that is approved by the FDA may be sold to any licensed physician, even though that physician may not have had any formal training in liposuction or any surgical credentials.

Your best chance for safe surgery and good outcomes begins by consulting with a plastic surgeon certified by the American Board of Plastic Surgery or a dermatologist certified by the American Board of Dermatology with added training in liposuction. Any provider you choose should have accredited training in liposuction, either in residency or through continuing education. No other providers have the specialized and appropriate training to perform liposuction for body contouring. Board-certified facial plastic surgeons with appropriate training in liposuction, as defined above, are appropriate providers for procedures of the face and neck.

Are you covered?

Liposuction for body contouring is an aesthetic procedure. When liposuction techniques are used in female breast reduction or other cases that may be considered reconstructive, insurance coverage may be provided. Check with your carrier and always obtain precertification.

Good candidates

Good candidates for liposuction of the body are individuals in good health, of good fitness, who are not excessively overweight and are not considering liposuction to be a means of weight control. Typically performed on adult men and women (although sometimes performed on some older adolescents), liposuction patients should be emotionally and physically healthy individuals who are bothered by the appearance of excess localized fat deposits.

In addition, as mentioned above, candidates for liposuction alone must have healthy skin with good elasticity. Also, individuals with health conditions that affect wound healing or bleeding, such as diabetes, anemia, edema, and blood clots, may not be good candidates. Individuals taking blood thinners, such as coumadin, persantine, or aspirin, may also be disqualified unless their medical physicians specifically say they may safely stop these medications during a given period before and after surgery.

> The American Society for Aesthetic Plastic Surgery reports in their 2003 procedural statistics that liposuction is the most common aesthetic procedure for both men and women, with just over 61,000 men undergoing liposuction in 2003, and just under 323,000 women having liposuction. This is a reported 117% increase in liposuction since 1997.

How it's done

Liposuction is a safe and immensely satisfying procedure for the right candidates when performed by qualified surgeons. Any liposuction technique requires first a careful evaluation of your physical condition including skin tone and the body contours that you wish to improve. Each individual is different in his or her physical shape. Therefore, each case of liposuction must be approached individually.

Prior to your surgery your surgeon will circle or mark the areas to be treated. (During the procedure, positioning, swelling, and fluids used in tumescent techniques will cause these areas to change in contour.)

If tumescent techniques are used, the areas to be suctioned will first be infiltrated with fluid. This numbs the area, constricts the blood vessels, and swells the fat cells. Once the area is distended or swollen (this defines tumescence) an appropriately sized cannula will be inserted through small, strategically placed

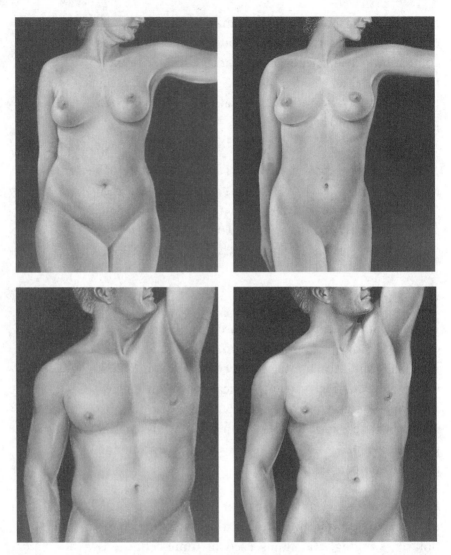

Figure 8   Liposuction before and after. This is an artist's rendering and does not represent actual patient results. Individual results may vary. Courtesy of the American Society of Plastic Surgeons®. All rights reserved. Learn more at *www.plasticsurgery.org*.

incisions. Once the cannula is below the surface of the skin and into a localized fat deposit, a controlled back-and-forth motion will loosen and suction subcutaneous fat to sculpt your new contours.

What to expect

Traditional liposuction is performed under general anesthesia or local anesthesia with sedation. Tumescent techniques include local anesthetic agents, and oral or intravenous sedation may be added for your comfort. Local anesthesia alone may be appropriate in more limited cases. Unless you have large-volume liposuction (defined in Question 53), the procedure will likely be performed on an out-patient basis in an office-based, ambulatory-, or hospital-based surgical setting.

Following the procedure, you will be uncomfortable and bruised in the areas that were suctioned. Discomfort may increase somewhat in the hours following surgery as anesthesia wears off and the healing process begins. Oral medications are generally adequate to control discomfort. If you have had ultra-sonic assisted liposuction (defined in Question 52), there may be small thin tubes placed in incisions to drain any excess fluid that might accumulate. You may be dressed in elastic bandages and a compression garment to help skin shrink back to your new smaller contours. Depending on your surgeon's preference, your incisions may or may not require stitches. In most cases only a stitch or two is required in each wound. Due to the amount of swelling and bandages it is unlikely you will see immediate results.

A responsible adult friend, family member, or caregiver will be required to be with you at all times for at least 24 hours following surgery. You will be encouraged to begin walking immediately following surgery to avoid the formation of blood clots. You will be encouraged to return to light normal activity as soon as possible and may shower as soon as your surgeon allows you to remove the compression garment and/or elastic bandages. Bicycle shorts or other lycra undergarments are helpful for support once the compression garment or elastic bandages are discontinued. Your surgeon will tell you when you may resume a more vigorous workout schedule.

What you need to know

Swelling and changes in sensation of the skin can be expected during your recovery. Complications include irregular contours that may require additional liposuction to revise. Pooling of liquid (hematoma or seroma) beneath the skin is also possible and may need to be drained. Fluid imbalance, infection, bleeding, shock, and pulmonary emboli are rare complications. Even more rare is the perforation of vital organs. Overdose of lidocaine with the fluid infusion of tumescent techniques has also been reported. The risk of serious complications is much higher when liposuction is performed in large volumes or when combined with other large and time-consuming procedures.

In consumer information on the safety of liposuction, the U.S. FDA cites studies that report death due to liposuction as low as 3 in 100,000 procedures.

Your responsibilities

Smokers will be required to stop smoking prior to surgery and throughout recovery. In addition, you may need to stop taking certain types of medications. You must follow all of your surgeon's instructions including wearing compression or support garments for as long as directed. The success of your outcome depends a great deal on your cooperation and compliance.

Maintaining a stable weight will increase the chances that the results of your liposuction will be long-lasting. (Pregnancy following liposuction of the abdomen may change your results, and you may want further surgery to correct sagging skin.)

Your goals

The final results of liposuction appear over time. Some changes will be visible immediately, and gradually your appearance will improve over several weeks as swelling and bruising subside. Depending on the areas suctioned and total fat removed, your final results will appear at about 6 months to 1 year.

Be sure to watch your weight following liposuction. Although fat is permanently removed, weight gain may cause the treated areas to become lumpy. This irregularity occurs because liposuction creates tunnels in the fat, it does not uniformly excise (remove by cutting out) all the cells in a given layer. Therefore, when you gain weight, the remaining cells get bigger in irregular numbers. Furthermore, you may find that you are developing fat pockets in areas you never thought existed, because fat cells in other areas are getting larger.

Revealing something new

The change in your body following liposuction may be small. Removal of the pooch of fat around the belly button may be all you desire. Or, you may wish to simply chisel away the rolls of fat at the waistline (love handles) on an otherwise trim and fit body. In other cases, you may desire much more extensive liposuction, and the results may be very dramatic. Thin young women with disproportionately large saddle-bags may lose as much as 2 to 3 pant sizes, not in the waist but in what was necessary to accommodate the girth of the thighs.

In any case, the new shape of your body following liposuction may lead you to engage in even more fitness and physical activity. You won't be as self-conscious about your body, and you may find yourself shopping for a new wardrobe. Not only might you need clothing in smaller sizes, you may want more fitted and revealing clothing now that your disproportionate fat has disappeared.

51. Is tumescent liposuction always used?

The tumescent technique offers multiple advantages over traditional liposuction, making it the current standard for liposuction. Developed by an American dermatologic surgeon, tumescent liposuction infuses areas to be suctioned with large volumes of local anesthetic agents and epinephrine, diluted in saline. When injected into the areas to be treated prior to suctioning, the fluid swells the fat cells, allowing them to be more easily suctioned. It also reduces the amount of your own body fluid that is lost during liposuction. The lidocaine numbs the area to be suctioned, increasing patient comfort and reducing the need for general anesthesia. The epinephrine constricts the blood vessels, resulting in less blood loss during surgery.

The benefits of liposuction using tumescent techniques far outweigh the only added risk: an overdose of lidocaine. This added risk is readily controlled by limiting the amount of fluid infiltrated to less than 5 liters in a single procedure.

52. What is ultrasound-assisted liposuction?

Ultrasound-assisted liposuction (UAL) uses ultrasonic (high-pitched sound) waves to loosen and melt fat cells prior to suctioning. It should never be performed on a patient with a pacemaker or any similar implanted device. UAL is generally performed after the area has been tumesced and is very helpful to treat certain areas of the body. In some cases UAL works to help shrink the skin to the newly formed contours. It is particularly advantageous where fatty tissue may be more fibrous such as in the back, male breast, the abdomen, and the hips.

There are added risks to liposuction with UAL. First there is the possibility of blistering or burning the skin where, from the inside out, the cannula pushes into the dermis (the deep side of the skin). Prior cannulas for internal UAL carried the risk of overheating and possibly causing internal burns. Newer instruments have shutoff mechanisms that reduce this risk. (Because it is not nearly as effective, external UAL is not greatly used. External UAL carries the added risk of thermal burns and scarring of the skin from the surface of the UAL device.)

53. What is large-volume liposuction?

Large-volume liposuction is defined as more than 5 liters of fat and fluid [or 5000 cubic centimeters (ccs)] removed during one procedure. The potential for significant fluid and electrolyte imbalances creating arrhythmias or shock is increased. Many patients can safely and successfully undergo large-volume liposuction under the care of an experienced surgeon. Overnight hospitalization or treatment in a special recovery facility to monitor patient health may be necessary.

While replacing lost fluids during any form of liposuction is essential to patient safety, infusing a patient with too much fluid carries risks of its own. Therefore, if you plan to have multiple large areas of excess fat removed, be certain that your surgeon is board certified and experienced in liposuction techniques; also, ensure that he or she can speak specifically to the special precautions necessary if large-volume liposuction is anticipated.

Generally, it is safer to perform liposuction in stages. The best results are achieved when the patient loses as much excess weight as possible first!

54. Is endermologie an alternative to liposuction?

Endermologie does not reduce excess fat. It is a procedure developed in France in the 1980s, originally designed to improve the condition of scars. It is essentially a form of mechanical massage with surface suction that can, in some cases, improve the physical condition of dimpled and uneven skin irregularities. In the United States endermologie is approved by the FDA for improvement of some scars and cellulite (the dimpled fat that occurs most commonly on the buttocks, hips, and thighs of some women). Endermologie requires multiple treatments, in some cases as many as 20 or more treatments to see improvement. As well, the results of endermologie are not permanent. When treatment is stopped some of the benefits of endermologie can be lost.

Endermologie is reported to reduce the circumference of the body in areas where cellulite is improved, but it does not in any way alter fat that exists below the skin's dermis. As much as liposuction cannot improve cellulite, endermologie is not a substitute for liposuction. If you really want to try endermologie, be prepared for a real time and money commitment before you see any visible results.

55. How can male breasts be reduced?

Gynecomastia is a condition defined as "woman-like breasts" in males. Gynecomastia is not always the result of obesity or a lack of fitness. Even men of exceptional fitness and ideal weight can have excessive breast tissue. Where it is caused by heredity, conditions usually begin at the onset of puberty. Other causes include the use of some medications such as prescription hormones, and the use of anabolic steroids or marijuana. Gynecomastia is not physically harmful to a man's health, but it can significantly affect emotional health, making men feel immensely self-conscious. Correction of gynecomastia reduces the curve and volume of a male breast and brings a masculine form to male breast contours. Gynecomastia may be corrected with liposuction or with surgical excision depending on the nature of the excessive breast tissue.

Are you covered?

Correction of gynecomastia is an aesthetic procedure that is not eligible for insurance coverage. The very rare exception is cases of severe and generally unilateral (or one-sided) gynecomastia, which some insurers may consider reconstructive; precertification is always required.

Good candidates

Good candidates for correction of gynecomastia are adolescent males whose breast size has been stable for more than two years. Fully grown men are also good candidates. But if there has been long-standing breast enlargement with stretching of the skin, the area will sag. Further procedures may be necessary to correct the skin.

Procedural specifics

Gynecomastia is corrected through one or both surgical techniques in body contouring:

- Surgical excision of tissue, and excess skin if necessary
- Liposuction

Good outcomes as well as your safety and satisfaction in treating gynecomastia require first carefully determining exactly what is causing the condition, that is, excess glandular tissue, fat, or both. For that reason, it is best to consult with a board-certified plastic surgeon with experience in both excision techniques and liposuction.

Where the condition is mostly dense glandular tissue, excision techniques may give the better outcome. Generally, incisions are concealed around the areola (the pigmented skin around the nipple) or in the underarm area. If excess skin is going to be removed, incisions will most likely be around the areola and sometimes in the breast crease. Incisions will require stitches. Special compression dressings may also be used.

Liposuction may be used in conjunction with excision where excess fat is a contributing factor of gynecomastia. Where only excess fat is a factor, liposuction alone may achieve the desired results. Tumescent and UAL techniques are appropriate. Read the questions about liposuction for complete information about these techniques.

What to expect

Surgery to correct gynecomastia will be performed under general anesthesia or local anesthesia with sedation; the type of anesthesia is dependent on the techniques used and your plastic surgeon's recommendations. In nearly every case it will be performed on an outpatient basis in an office-, ambulatory-, or hospital-based surgical facility. Following surgery you will likely be sore, somewhat swollen, and possibly bruised. You may have an elastic bandage wrapped around your chest to compress the skin to your new body contours and to support tissue as it heals. Small, thin tubes may be placed in your incisions to drain any excess fluid. Discomfort should be controlled with oral medications. Most importantly, you must have a responsible adult, a family member, friend, or caregiver to stay with you for at least 24 hours following surgery even though you may feel fully capable of caring for yourself.

You will be able to resume light normal activity as soon as possible as long as you don't do any heavy lifting, pushing, or pulling. Within 1 to 2 weeks, stitches used to close your incisions may be removed. Depending on the techniques used and the extent of your procedure, you should be able to engage in regular daily activity as soon as you feel ready. Any physical activity that requires heavy lifting or use of your upper body strength should be avoided until healing is full completed and as directed by your plastic surgeon.

What you need to know

Risks and complications from correction of gynecomastia include the possibility of blood loss, pooling of blood or fluid beneath the skin, poor healing of incisions, infection, and all the risks associated with liposuction if liposuction techniques were used. In addition, there are risks associated with anesthesia.

Irregular contours and asymmetry are possible. Perfect symmetry between the breasts is not always possible. In addition, surgery to revise unsatisfactory outcomes or excision of excess skin may need to be performed to improve your results.

Your responsibilities

Foremost, you are responsible for following all of your surgeon's instructions, including cessation of smoking before surgery and throughout recovery. Wound care and activity instructions must be understood and carefully followed. If your condition was caused by the use of anabolic steroids or marijuana, consider quitting altogether, not only for the sake of your appearance, but also for your health.

Your goals

The results of gynecomastia surgery are visible immediately, although they will not be fully achieved until all swelling has diminished. The results of correction of gynecomastia are generally permanent. However, excessive weight gain can, in some cases, change male breast contours. In addition, when gynecomastia correction is performed on adolescents whose growth is not fully completed, additional growth may change the results.

More than physical

An increase in male confidence is likely to occur almost immediately following correction of gynecomastia. Some men may find themselves more motivated than ever to be fit. To adolescents and young adult males, the correction of gynecomastia may also bring improved social skills and even improved performance at school. Confidence is greatly enhanced when what may have been the source of extreme ridicule and shame no longer exits. Form-fitting T-shirts, sweaters, and swim trunks will be among many new additions to your wardrobe.

> The American Society for Aesthetic Plastic Surgery (ASAPS) in 2003 reported over 22,000 procedures to correct gyncomastia. This is a distinct decline from past years as reported by the ASPS, nearly 28% since 2000. Why such a reduction? Most likely many men are turning to newer liposuction techniques and receiving treatment in more than one area. Thus, the procedure is simply recorded as liposuction, of which nearly 16% of patients were men according to ASAPS in 2003.

56. How is a bulging tummy corrected?

A tummy tuck, also called abdominoplasty, improves the contours of the abdominal area to produce a flatter, more toned appearance. Tummy tuck corrects more than a bulge; in cases where your waistline has disappeared or folds over, a tummy tuck can produce a flatter, more trimmed abdomen. Tummy tuck is not a substitute for fitness or weight loss. The procedure corrects excess skin in the abdomen and may tighten the abdominal muscles. It may also remove a small amount of fat. The conditions suitable for treatment with abdominoplasty may:

- Be localized to the lower or central abdomen
- Involve the entire abdomen
- Involve the entire abdomen and extend to the back

In addition to correcting excess skin and fat in the abdomen, a tummy tuck can also correct a condition called diastasis, a vertical separation of the abdominal wall muscle that especially occurs in some women following pregnancy.

There are varying degrees to the conditions that are corrected by tummy tuck and therefore varying techniques to achieve desired outcomes. Where only excess fat is the contributing factor and skin has good tone and elasticity, liposuction techniques alone may achieve good results. (Be sure to read the questions about liposuction.) This is not called a tummy tuck, but it is liposuction of the abdomen.

A true tummy tuck treats excess abdominal skin (or "apron") and requires surgical excision of skin to create a flatter, more trimmed tummy. Anyone who is considering a tummy tuck should meet with a board-certified plastic surgeon to determine exactly what procedures will achieve the best overall outcome.

Are you covered?

Tummy tuck is an aesthetic procedure. In cases where abdominal overhand is so excessive that it causes back problems and skin infections, the repair of certain associated areas may be covered by insurance. Hernias may also be covered. Precertification is necessary in these instances.

Good candidates

Tummy tuck candidates are healthy men and women with excess abdominal skin who are of stable weight and not obese. They are individuals with realistic goals

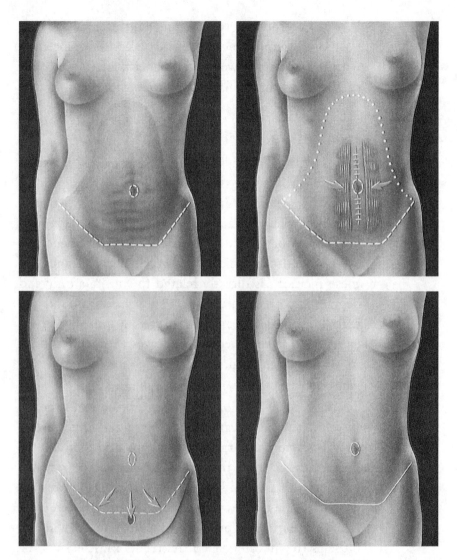

Figure 9 "Tummy tuck" (abdominoplasty). This is an artist's rendering and does not represent actual patient results. Individual results may vary.

who do not have health conditions that can impede healing, such as diabetes or certain autoimmune diseases. If you have a condition that may compromise your health, make certain your plastic surgeon and your primary care physician communicate.

Women considering future pregnancies may wish to postpone a tummy tuck. Tummy tuck will not interfere with pregnancy; however, the benefits of tummy tuck can be significantly diminished following pregnancy.

How it's done

The tummy tuck is performed by excision of excess skin (and sometime the removal of fat) through incisions. In general, tummy tuck incisions are placed above the pubic bone. Incisions can be as short as a few inches or extend from hipbone to hipbone (and even around the back). The length and placement of these incisions is directly related to your anatomy and degree of correction needed. An incision around the belly button will be made except in a mini-lift where excess skin is confined to the lower abdomen and no muscle repair is required.

Through these incisions skin and subcutaneous (below the skin) fat are elevated from the underlying muscles and dissection is carried to the ribs and sternum. A hole is cut around the belly button, and it remains attached to its blood supply. Deep internal sutures are used to shape the new abdominal contours where necessary. If diastasis is present, your separated abdominal muscles (technically called the rectus muscles) will be repositioned and rejoined. After any excess fat is removed and internal corrections are made, the skin is pulled downward toward the incision. Excess tissue is then trimmed away and the incisions are closed with stitches or metal clips. A new opening for your belly button will be made, and the belly button will be sutured to the edges of the hole.

What to expect

Tummy tuck is commonly, although not always, performed under general anesthesia. Whether or not an overnight stay in a hospital or special recovery facility is recommended depends upon the extent of surgery required. In most cases, tummy tuck can be performed in an office-, ambulatory-, or hospital-based surgical facility.

During the first 24 to 48 hours following recovery it is imperative that a responsible, alert adult friend, family member, or caregiver be with you at all times, depending on the extent of your surgery. You will experience some tightness and discomfort in the abdominal area as well as at the incision sites. This can be controlled with medication.

In most cases, you will be advised by your plastic surgeon not to stand upright and to sleep only in a reclining position with pillows supporting the knees, generally for 1 to 2 weeks following surgery. You may also need assistance with basic functions such as dressing and going to the bathroom for the first few days. It is imperative that you begin walking as soon as possible to reduce the chance of blood clot formation.

You may have small thin tubes placed to drain any excess fluid that accumulates. You may also be wrapped in an elastic bandage or simply have dressings around your incisions. Light normal activity is possible as soon as you feel ready.

External sutures or metal clips will likely be removed within one to two weeks. Your abdominal tissues might feel firm for some time as healing progresses, and you will be numb. Most swelling should subside within 2 to 4 months, with more final results taking 6 months to a year. Your incision sites will continue to soften, fade, and improve over the next 1 to 2 years. The scars from a tummy tuck are permanent as they are with any surgery. But placement of scars is easily concealed by most briefs, panties, and swimsuit bottoms.

What you need to know

Tummy tuck is a very safe procedure when performed by a qualified plastic surgeon on an appropriately healthy candidate. Asymmetry is a possible outcome. Infection, blood clots, pooling of blood beneath the skin, excess fluid accumulation, loss of tissue (necrosis), and, in rare cases, pulmonary emboli are possible. The formation of raised or irregular scars is also possible. In addition, there are risks of injuring the abdominal tissue if you try to stand upright before adequate healing. As with any surgery, there may be a need for minor revisions, and there are the risks associated with anesthesia.

Your responsibilities

Smoking can greatly impair healing, and therefore it is essential that you stop smoking for several weeks prior to surgery and throughout your recovery. In addition, you must follow all of your surgeon's instructions precisely. While it may be uncomfortable to stand only in a flexed position for several days, this is imperative to your healing and to achieving a good outcome. Your advantage to having scars that heal well is through proper wound care and by following all instructions for use of topical ointments, silicone sheeting, and massage of the incision sites.

In addition, you must maintain a stable, healthy weight and resume regular exercise to retain the improvement a tummy tuck brings to your abdomen and the appearance of your body.

Your goals

In general, the results of tummy tuck are permanent, although these results can change with aging and/or fluctuations in weight. Healthy eating and regular exercise will only enhance the outcomes of your procedure. Once the excess apron of tissue hanging from your abdomen is replaced by a smooth, toned tummy and visible waistline, you may want new clothing. And you may find a new freedom to engage in more physical activities and new confidence to bare just a little more.

The number of tummy tucks performed in the United States in 2003 was over 101,000 as reported by the American Society of Plastic Surgeons. Of this, 6% of patients were men, with a steady rise in the number of procedures and male patients over recent years.

57. How can a sagging, flabby body appearance be corrected?

Body lifts are surgical procedures performed to correct excess loose, sagging skin and underlying fat that exists anywhere in the torso and extremities. (Tummy tuck is a surgical body lift procedure, specific to the abdominal area, see Question 56.) A body lift reshapes the body contours and removes sagging skin.

Surgical body lifts correct conditions that result from aging, weight loss, and multiple pregnancies (with the associated weight gain and loss). In some cases, the

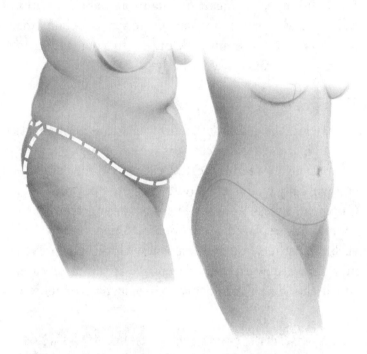

Figure 10. Body lift. This is an artist's rendering and does not represent actual patient results. Individual results may vary.

conditions that are corrected by body lifts may be hereditary: familial fat deposits and skin that lacks tone and elasticity. Surgical body lifts can result in a dramatic improvement in the condition and appearance of your contours and skin. (Brachioplasty, or lift of the upper arm, will be discussed specifically in Question 58).

Are you covered?

Body lifts are aesthetic procedures. There may be exceptions in cases where body-lifting techniques are performed to reconstruct the body where excess hanging skin is causing medical problems such as macerated (wet) skin that frequently becomes infected. In these cases precertification for insurance coverage is necessary.

Good candidates

Body lift candidates are healthy men and women who are not obese and where weight is stable. They are individuals with realistic goals who are willing to accept that the trade-off for a better body contour is the presence of visible scars.

If you have health conditions that can impede healing, such as diabetes or certain autoimmune diseases, you may not be a good candidate for a body lift. It is important that you disclose any condition that may compromise your health, and you need to have your plastic surgeon and primary care physician communicate if there are health issues.

Women who are planning future pregnancies may be advised to postpone a body lift. The results of a body lift can be significantly diminished following pregnancy, especially if there is more than the recommended weight gain.

How it's done

Body lifts should only be performed by plastic surgeons certified by the American Board of Plastic Surgery, who have experience in this growing segment of body contouring procedures. Your plastic surgeon will fully evaluate your condition, and then determine how to best achieve your goals. In fact, your body lift may not be performed at one time, but staged over more than one surgical session.

Prior to body lift, your plastic surgeon will likely mark incision patterns and areas to be treated. The scars from these incisions are permanent, but newer techniques will allow your scars to be concealed by modest undergarments. Every lower body lift incision pattern is individualized to the patient; however, there are three more common pattern formations:

- A thong bikini outline incision pattern with a full incision around the waist is common for a full lower body lift, allowing the thighs, hips, and buttocks to be treated as well as the abdomen, waist, and lower back. A belt of excess fat and tissue is removed from around the waistline, as well as in a thong pattern on the buttocks.
- The waist, abdomen, groin, and upper thigh can be treated with a lateral tension abdominal lift with incisions of a traditional scooped bikini pattern only on the front of the body. This technique does not produce any lift in the buttocks or in the back of the thighs.
- The buttocks and thighs alone can be treated with an incision pattern at the crease of the buttocks.

Liposuction techniques maybe used in conjunction with body lift. Then excess tissue will be undermined (elevated) or excised (cut out) and the underlying deep tissue forming body contours will be "lifted" or smoothed toward the incisions and into a new shape or contour. These stitches are either dissolving or permanent; they will not be removed. Excess skin is also lifted or smoothed upward or downward, and any further excess skin is removed. The incisions are closed with stitches or metal clips.

What to expect

Body lift procedures are most commonly performed under general anesthesia. The procedure can be performed on an outpatient basis in an office-, ambulatory-, or hospital-based surgical setting. Depending on the extent of your procedure and your plastic surgeon's recommendations, you may be advised to have an overnight stay in a hospital or a special recovery facility to carefully monitor your progress following surgery.

When you awaken from surgery, you may be wrapped in elastic bandages to minimize swelling and help support your new body contours as they heal. Small thin tubes may be placed to drain any excess fluid that accumulates. Your incision sites may be uncomfortable, and your lower body will be sore. The discomfort can usually be controlled with medication prescribed by your plastic surgeon.

You will not be able to stand fully upright, nor should you try. You may need to use a walker or crutches to support you when you walk for the first week following surgery. You will be encouraged to walk immediately to minimize the possibility of forming blood clots. If you will recover fully at home, a responsible adult will be required to be with you at all times for at least the first 48 hours following surgery. You may need assistance in basic functions such as getting up and going to the bathroom.

You will need to rest for several days following surgery, with light walking as part of your postoperative regimen. If abdominoplasty (tummy tuck) is included in your procedure, you will be walking in a slightly angled or bent over position. When resting, you will need to remain in a reclining position; placing pillows under your knees is also helpful. If you have incisions on your buttocks, an inflatable cushion may be helpful to keep the pressure off those incisions when you are reclining or sitting. Within one to two weeks, you should be standing upright and walking without any assistance. At this time you will be ready to resume normal daily activities.

What you need to know

The risks and complications of body lift procedures are carefully controlled when under the care of a board-certified plastic surgeon experienced with body lift. However, complications are always possible and include hematoma (an accumulation of blood or fluid underneath the skin), embolism, infection, nerve damage, and necrosis (loss of healthy tissue). In addition, there is also the risk of excessive or raised and firm scars, and as with any surgery there are risks associated with anesthesia. In cases where irregular contours develop or where your results are not fully achieved, you may need additional surgery to revise your outcomes.

Your responsibilities

Following all of your plastic surgeon's instructions precisely before surgery is essential to your safety. It is also important to follow all postoperative instructions, including activity restrictions and requirements for proper wound care.

Your goals

Body lift results are immediate, although they will be obscured by swelling and bandages. In addition, soft tissue will refine and settle into the newly shaped contours over time. The very firm feeling you have in the surgical areas will soften over many months following surgery.

Stitches will likely be removed within 1 to 2 weeks. Massaging of the scars, wearing compression or silicone tape, and applying certain ointments will aid in refining scars. Scars are permanent and will always be visible. Scar placement and length should be of no surprise to you; your plastic surgeon should have fully explained and illustrated potential scars to you prior to surgery.

You will usually be able to resume normal fitness within 4 to 6 weeks following surgery. Maintaining your results requires that you adhere to a healthy lifestyle of proper diet and exercise. As long as your weight does not significantly change, your lower body lift results should last many years. Your body will not age as quickly as it would had you not undergone body lift surgery.

The trade-off

You will probably want new clothing to flatter your newly shaped firmer, slimmer, and more-toned body contours. With the confidence you gain, you may feel ready to wear a swimsuit or shorts again, and to engage in more athletic and fitness activities. However, you will have very long scars that are necessary to have achieved your body lift. In many cases your scars can be concealed by modest undergarments. But in all cases they are permanent, and you must be willing to accept this as the trade-off to your new improved body contour.

> Surgical lower body lifts have been popular in Europe and Latin American for many years, but advances by U.S. doctors have made the procedure safer and more desirable. According to reported statistics by the American Society for Aesthetic Plastic Surgery, lower body lift procedures numbered nearly 11,000 in 2003.

58. Can body lifts correct sagging, droopy arms?

An upper arm lift, or brachioplasty, is a surgical lift of the upper arm. It corrects the loose and flabby tissue that results in a very saggy batwing-like appearance of the back of the upper arm. The procedure reduces excess skin and fat in the upper arm to create a smoother, toned contour of the triceps area. Upper arm lift does not, however, improve muscle tone, which is something that requires regular, focused exercise. Upper arm lift is for individuals who have lost significant weight, who have hereditary fat deposits at the back of the arm, or who have very good muscle tone but have lost skin elasticity. The results can present a very remarkable improvement in the appearance, shape, and tone of the upper arm. The results also include a permanent and visible scar inside the upper arm and/or axilla (underarm).

Are you covered?

Brachioplasty is not covered by insurance, as it is an aesthetic procedure. There may be exceptions in cases where a brachioplasty is performed to reconstruct the body where excess hanging skin is causing medical problems such as macerated (wet, easily infected) skin. If this is the case, precertification for insurance coverage is necessary.

Good candidates

Brachioplasty candidates are healthy men and women who are of stable weight and not obese. If you have health conditions that can impede healing, such as diabetes or severe autoimmune disease, you may not be a good candidate for brachioplasty. Your best option is to disclose any condition that may compromise your health, and to have your plastic surgeon and primary care physician communicate.

How it's done

An upper arm lift, like any surgical procedure involving aesthetic shaping of the body, should only be performed by a plastic surgeon certified by the American Board of Plastic Surgery. In some cases, liposuction techniques may be performed in conjunction with upper arm lift to remove localized excess fat in the upper arm.

The procedure requires an incision generally beginning in the curve of the underarm area (axilla) that extends outward and downward on the inside of the upper arm. The length, size, and placement of the incision depend on the degree of correction needed to achieve a smooth and even contour of the upper arm. In cases where more limited correction is required, an incision in the axilla (or underarm area) and/or a smaller incision along the upper inner arm may be used. Through the incision, sagging loose underlying tissues will be reshaped and tightened with any excess tissue removed. Deep nonremovable sutures will hold the new contours of these deeper tissues in place. The skin is then smoothed inward with excess skin carefully trimmed away and outside incisions closed with stitches.

What to expect

When performed alone, brachioplasty is an outpatient procedure performed under local anesthesia with sedation or under general anesthesia, in your plastic surgeon's office-, ambulatory-, or hospital-based surgical facility.

When your arm lift surgery is complete, you may have your arms wrapped in elastic bandages to support your new contours during initial healing. You may have a small thin tube placed to drain any excess fluid that accumulates. Your arms will likely be stiff and very sore or achy, and may be swollen. This is normal, and any pain or discomfort can usually be controlled with medication. You will be released to the care of an adult family member, friend, or caregiver who must remain with you at all times for at least 24 hours following surgery. You will need assistance, as raising your arms even a small amount may be uncomfortable. You should not attempt to hold anything heavy.

Your discomfort should subside quickly and you should resume light normal activity right away, as long as you do not use your arms for any physical activity that is highly uncomfortable or strenuous in any way.

What you need to know

Risks and complications of brachioplasty are carefully controlled when you are under the care of a board-certified plastic surgeon experienced with the procedure. However, complications are always possible and include hematoma (an accumulation of blood or fluid underneath the skin), embolism, infection, nerve damage, and necrosis (loss of tissue). In addition, there is also the risk of excessive or raised and firm scars, and as with any surgery, there are risks associated with anesthesia. In cases where irregular contours develop or where your results are not fully achieved, you may need additional surgery to revise your outcomes.

Your responsibilities

Following all of your plastic surgeon's directions regarding cessation of smoking, medications, wound care, and activity is essential to a good outcome. If you engage in too strenuous an activity, you could risk bleeding, opening of the wound, thickening of scars, and a poor outcome.

Your goals

The results of surgical upper arm lift are visible immediately and will continue to improve as swelling subsides and incisions heal. Your stitches will be removed within a week or two. You may be given ointment or compression tapes to help scars further improve. However, scars are permanent and visible on the inside of the upper arm.

The stiffness and soreness in your arms will improve quickly after the first few weeks. You may resume normal daily activity at this time, including the full use of your arms. Within 4 to 6 weeks you should be back to complete normal physical activity and even lifting heavier weight with your arms.

Well armed

An upper arm lift offers immensely satisfying and safe results to correct a baggy, droopy upper arm. You will find that clothing fits better and, despite visible scars, you may want to wear short sleeves or even go sleeveless. The physical condition of the triceps muscle has little to do with the conditions of the skin of the upper arm that is corrected by a lift. However, it is still advised that you practice regular, targeted exercises to keep the muscles in the upper arms strong and toned. Exercise can only improve your outcomes from surgical arm lift.

The American Society for Aesthetic Plastic Surgery reports nearly 11,000 upper arm lift procedures in 2003. Until 2000, data on these procedures were not regularly collected.

59. How can I improve my sagging skin following major weight loss?

Recontouring following major weight loss (such as with bariatric or gastric bypass surgery) can result in a small or great amount of all-over excess sagging, and loose skin and tissue.

The first consideration before undergoing any surgical procedure following weight loss is that the

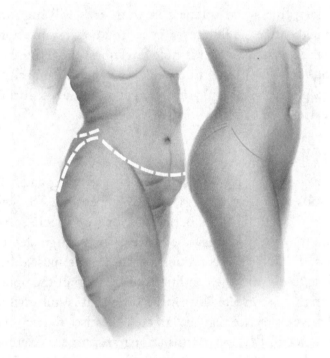

Figure 11. This is an artist's rendering and does not represent actual patient results. Individual results may vary.

weight loss is complete and stabilized. Further weight loss can greatly diminish the results, and rapid weight gain can present very unpleasant conditions, such as stretchmarks and poorly healed, wide scars. Patients undergoing recontouring procedures following weight loss need to accept the trade-off of firmer skin and smooth body contours for long visible scars. These scars result from the incisions necessary to reduce excess skin and to tighten underlying tissues that sag.

Are you covered?

At present there are no standards for insurance coverage for such recontouring. If you have had bariatric or gastric bypass surgery, you should check with your insurer for policies on coverage of recontouring procedures and always obtain precertification where coverage may be available.

Good candidates

Good candidates are those men and women whose weight loss is complete and stabilized, and who do not have any dangerous health conditions. You should have a positive outlook and be willing to accept all the conditions, stages, and trade-offs that body contouring surgeries will demand. You must be ready for a large physical, emotional, and financial investment. It may take several stages to achieve your final outcome.

How it's done

Recontouring following weight loss should only be performed by a plastic surgeon who is board-certified and experienced in liposuction and surgical body contouring techniques.

The conditions corrected through recontouring following major weight loss develop as follows: with initial weight gain, the fat cells increase in size, thereby stretching out the skin. With subsequent weight loss, the fat cells shrink, but severely stretched skin may not fully conform to the new smaller body contour. The result is excess loose and sagging skin. This commonly occurs in the cheeks, jowls, and neck; in the breast region, underarm, and upper arm; in the waistline and abdomen; and in the thighs, hips, buttocks, and groin. Body lifting reshapes supportive underlying tissue and removes excess skin. In some cases liposuction may also be used to remove irregular fatty deposits.

Each patient undergoing recontouring following major weight loss has his or her own set of deformities that need to be addressed. In most cases, it is best to undergo recontouring in stages. Overly long procedures and procedures requiring a great deal of patient repositioning may result in increased complications. Your plastic surgeon will recommend a strategic plan for your recontouring with which you both should be comfortable.

Procedures that may be included in your plan for recontouring are facelift, a breast lift, brachioplasty, abdominoplasty, and other body lifts.

What to expect

What you should expect is a lengthy consultation to evaluate your condition and understand your goals for improvement. Then you and your plastic surgeon can plan the course of your recontouring in stages. Usually, similar anatomic areas are treated together in the most practical way. For instance, the abdomen may be treated at the same time as the inner thighs. Buttocks and outer thighs are treated together and may be performed at the same time as the inner thigh or abdomen. Treatment of the upper body may be coupled with treatment of the arms. The face and neck may be treated in another surgical session. Once a plan for your recontouring is defined, specifically note the procedures your plastic surgeon recommends and the incision patterns he or she diagrams. Then carefully review all the sections of this chapter as well as facelift and breast lift if these relate to your case.

What you need to know

The risks and complications of recontouring following major weight loss include all of those risk and complications for each of the specific procedures you will undergo: body lifts, brachioplasty or arm lift, breast lift, facelift, and possibly liposuction. This includes the possibility of hematoma (an accumulation of blood or fluid underneath the skin), embolism, infection, nerve damage, and necrosis (loss of healthy tissue). In addition, there is also the risk of excessive or raised and firm scars, and as with any surgery there are risks associated with anesthesia. There is also the risk of asymmetry or uneven contours that will require additional surgery to revise your outcomes.

The added caution is that your body has been though massive physical and metabolic changes. This requires you to be physically and emotionally healthy enough to withstand the further changes resulting from your surgical treatments.

Your responsibilities

Your responsibilities include following all of your plastic surgeon's instructions carefully. Recontouring following major weight loss may take nearly as much time as the weight loss itself. Giving yourself enough time for healing between stages is imperative. You must be patient—it's worth it.

Your goals

Bariatric and gastric bypass procedures have become much more available and may have been the catalyst in your goal to lose weight. Although the weight loss was necessary for you to achieve a new body size, treatment of the resulting sagging tissues will achieve your new contours.

Various lifts will refine your body, tone, and overall appearance both in and out of clothing. Most individuals who have undergone these procedures following major weight loss are often more excited about the results of plastic surgery than they were about the weight loss itself. The trade-off of the resulting scars may well be worth the changes you will see in your appearance. The results of recontouring are permanent as long as your weight remains stable.

60. Are there other forms of body contouring?

Most people undergo body contouring to slim and tone. But there are procedures in body contouring that augment, or actually enhance, the curves and shape of the body. Female breast augmentation with implants is one procedure, more appropriately classified as a plastic surgery of the breast and fully discussed in Part 7. Other forms of augmentation in body contouring that use a form of implant to enhance the body contours include pectoral or male chest augmentation, buttock augmentation, calf augmentation, and bicep and tricep augmentation. These procedures are designed to enhance the contour and appearance of muscular structures of the body where exercise cannot achieve desired results, most commonly due to heredity. Unlike breast augmentation implants that are fluid-filled silicone rubber shells, the implants used in these body augmentation procedures are made of medical-grade solid silicone rubber.

Are you covered?

Muscle or body augmentation with implants is an aesthetic procedure. Only in rare cases where the defect is due to trauma or disease might reimbursement be possible. Precertification is required.

Good candidates

Good candidates for body contouring by augmentation are healthy, very fit individuals who are willing to accept that these procedures can produce improvement, not perfection, and who are willing to accept the risks associated with this form of implant surgery.

How it's done

Only a very small percentage of board-certified plastic surgeons in the United States currently practice muscular augmentation for body contouring with implants. Because of the very unique nature of these procedures and the risks involved, make certain any plastic surgeon with whom you consult has ample experience with body implants. He or she should be explicit about the very specific considerations and risks you must accept before undergoing augmentation with these implants.

Body contouring with implants of the pectoral, bicep, tricep, buttock, or calf muscles requires surgical placement of specially formed solid-silicone implants. Implants will be placed through incisions in a pocket generally made below the skin and actual muscle to be augmented. Incisions will be closed with stitches. The following are the usual incision placement areas for body contouring implants:

- Buttocks: in the lower curve/crease of the buttocks
- Pectoral: at the areola (pigmented skin surrounding the nipple), in the underarm, or in the lower breast contour
- Calf: behind the knee
- Bicep: in the crease of the elbow
- Tricep: in the underarm

What to expect

Body contouring with implants is almost always performed under general anesthesia, and on an outpatient basis either in your plastic surgeon's office-based surgical facility, or in an ambulatory or hospital surgical facility. Once the procedure is completed you will awaken to find the surgical site sore, tight, and, in many cases, swollen. You will likely have the surgical area wrapped in a compression garment or elastic bandages to support the soft tissue and muscle as it heals around the implant.

You will be very stiff and sore for several days following surgery; discomfort can be controlled with medication. During those initial days of healing, also expect the following:

- Buttock implants: It will be uncomfortable to sit, lay on your back or walk.
- Calf implants: Walking will be uncomfortable.

- Pectoral, bicep, or tricep implant: Lifting, carrying anything, or raising your arms will be difficult and uncomfortable.

Stitches will usually be removed in a week or two following surgery, and you may be required to wear the bandages or compression for some time until healing is fully completed.

What you need to know

Risks with implants for body contouring include infection around the implant or at the incision sites. The implants may shift or extrude (be forced out to the surface), leaving large scars. Irregularly firm scar tissue may form around the implant, and external scars may thicken. In some cases the implants may need to be replaced or removed. In addition, as with any surgery there are associated risks of bleeding and fluid accumulation, nerve damage, and the risks of anesthesia. Further, the placement or removal of these implants may cause permanent muscle damage or disfigurement.

Your obligations

Patients must follow all instructions provided by their surgeon precisely, in order to enhance their opportunity for good outcomes. Excessive or improper movement during the initial phases of healing could cause the implant to shift. Additional surgery will be required to correct this shift.

Your goals

The outcome in your appearance following body contouring to augment muscular contours is visible almost immediately. The results are permanent, as long as the implants do not shift or need to be removed for any reason. Many individuals cannot achieve proportionate body contours due to small or irregular muscle development, despite vigorous efforts. For these patients, the improvement possible with body implants can be very fulfilling.

Dis-figuring

Although augmentation with body implants, namely buttock implants, may be a trend in some places, the decision to have these implants should not be impulsive. The results of this type of augmentation will affect you for life. If the implants need to be removed and you choose not to replace them, the resulting appearance may be very different from your preoperative contour. Tissues may sag, and a body lift may be required for an improved contour.

The American Society for Aesthetic Plastic Surgery reported the following in 2003: 3,385 buttock augmentation procedures (nearly 5 times the number of procedures performed in 2002), 1,734 male chest or pectoral augmentations (more than twice that of 2002), and 1,170 calf augmentations (over 6 times the number of procedures reported in 2002). Calf augmentation was the least reported of all aesthetic surgical procedures. The American Society of Plastic Surgeons did not report on buttock, pectoral, or calf augmentation as of 2003.

PART NINE

Beauty and Balance: Plastic Surgery to Change Facial Structure

What is plastic surgery of the facial structure?

What are rhinoplasty, facial implants, and otoplasty?

Can children have facial plastic surgery safely?

More . . .

Plastic surgery to alter the facial structures most commonly includes changing the shape, angles, and proportions of the face, nose, and ears. Some procedures are aesthetic, meaning that they are performed to improve appearance. Other procedures are reconstructive in nature and include surgery after tumor removal, after trauma, and repair of congenital anomalies (such as a cleft lip and palate). This category of facial surgery includes children, teens, and adults as appropriate candidates.

61. What is facial structural surgery?

Facial structure is determined primarily by bone and cartilage; facial appearance is determined by facial structure as well as overlying soft tissues (muscle, fat, and skin). Facial structural change is plastic surgery that reshapes bone and cartilage as well as the overlying soft tissues. Surgical techniques or the use of implants improve the size, shape, angle, or contour of the nose, chin, jaw, ears, and cheeks.

Facial structural surgery can produce very subtle to very dramatic changes in appearance. But before undergoing any surgery, you need to accept that altering your appearance will not change your life, or deny your genetic or ethnic origin. It may, however, give you a greater degree of self-confidence.

Understand that the results of plastic surgery to change facial structures are permanent and can only be modified through additional surgical procedures. Therefore, you must be confident in your desire for a given change in your facial structure as well as in the surgeon you choose and his or her recommended course of treatment.

Reconstructive and aesthetic plastic surgery for children requires the child's input in the decision-making process, whenever possible. No procedure that is aesthetic in nature should be forced upon a child who is able to comprehend medical treatment and care. A child should be able to understand what surgery or treatment can achieve, what he or she will experience, and what is expected of him or her during the course of care and recovery. A child should be able to fully express his or her feelings about having surgery and be psychologically prepared as much as possible.

The most common facial structural surgery is nose surgery (rhinoplasty). In addition, facial implants and ear surgery are frequently performed aesthetic plastic surgery procedures. Many of these procedures may be performed for reconstructive purposes to restore a more normal appearance or to restore function (such as rhinoplasty after nasal fracture). Facial structural surgery also can enhance rejuvenative surgeries, those that restore a more youthful appearance (such as a chin implant with a face lift).

62. Are there special considerations for children?

Plastic surgery of the facial structures is one category of procedures where children and adolescents may be good candidates. Plastic surgery may be recommended for children as young as infancy to correct a congenital or birth defect of the face. For example, repair of a cleft lip and/or palate can begin as early as 10 weeks of age. Repair of microtia (an absence or incomplete formation of the outer ear) may begin at one year of age.

The most common pediatric plastic surgery procedure of the facial structures is otoplasty (surgery to correct a protruding ear). The appropriate age, course of treatment, and support systems need to be addressed using a team approach. The child and his or her parents (or guardians), pediatrician, and plastic surgeon should work together to create a strategic plan for surgery. The team approach is important for most pediatric plastic surgeries to create a smooth recovery and to prevent developmental or emotional damage to a small

Beauty and Balance

Consistently in 2003 and the seven years prior, board-certified plastic surgeons performed 40,000 to 44,000 procedures each year to reconstruct birth defects, as reported by the American Society of Plastic Surgeons.

The American Society of Plastic Surgeons reports nearly 27,000 ear surgery procedures in 2003 performed both on children and adults.

The American Academy of Pediatrics offers information on choosing a pediatric plastic surgeon that can be downloaded from: http://www.aap. org/sections/ plassurg.htm.

child. In cases of extensive surgeries, psychologists, neurologists, dentists, and other professionals may need to be part of the team as well.

A parent or guardian must make the final decision for plastic surgery. When surgery is to be performed primarily for aesthetic purposes, there are many issues that need to be considered. First, talk to your child. Allow her or him to communicate the hopes of what surgery can accomplish. For example, a child may not state, "I wish my ears didn't stick out." But he or she may ask, "Why do people say I have Dumbo ears?" The ridicule of peers may not justify, to you, the decision for surgery. But if you see changes in your child's personality or signs of depression (withdrawal, changing sleep patterns, changing eating habits), communication is crucial.

A child must also be able understand and accept the experiences associated with surgery. You and your surgeon must carefully discuss the realities of surgery with your child in a manner he or she can fully understand, but without alarm. You must express that there are certain expectations of your child following surgery, too, such as restricted activity and keeping bandages in place. You must feel confident that your child will be cooperative. Most importantly, you must feel confident in your child's desire to have surgery and in the provider you have chosen.

One note: We have discussed that patients should not expect plastic surgery to dramatically change their lives. From an adult perspective, this is certainly true. But from the perspective of a child who has felt shamed or been subjected to ridicule related to his or her appearance, plastic surgery can indeed be a life-changing event. The shy, reserved child who avoided interaction with others may suddenly blossom into an outgoing and social individual. Some children may even improve in their performance at school. And, what was once a negative or uncooperative child may become a very positive, productive, and pleasant one.

Teenaged children obsess about appearance, clothing, and image. It is a rite of passage that just about every parent of a teen has seen. While their behavior may seem impulsive, many adolescents have legitimate reasons to want to undergo plastic surgery and are, in fact, good candidates.

Plastic surgery can vastly improve self-esteem in cases where appearance makes a teen feel physically inadequate. If an adolescent states on multiple occasions that he or she wants a specific surgery, a thorough discussion may be in order. No pressure from outside influences (including family and friends) should force a teen's decision. However, the support of family and friends is vital. A teen should not only be able to express desire, but also define—specifically—what he or she wishes to correct and why. He or she should have realistic expectations regarding the outcomes of surgery with respect to appearance, and also on quality of life.

A trusted and supportive adult must accompany a teen, no matter how responsible that teen is, to consult with a plastic surgeon. The plastic surgeon can then more easily assess motivations and maturity, and thereby determine whether the teen is, indeed, a good candidate for a given procedure.

63. What is facial harmony?

Facial harmony is not a musical term; it describes the relative proportion and balance of facial features. Components of facial harmony include (among other things) the size, contours, and angles of the ears, nose, cheek, forehead, jaw, and chin. Facial features that are proportionate to one another create facial harmony—no one feature is significantly more prominent or different in appearance than the others.

Where a lack of facial harmony exists, the offending features are generally readily identified. However, achieving facial harmony does not always mean correction of the offending or disproportionate features. For example, a patient with a very high and broad forehead that is disproportionate to relatively normal features may achieve facial harmony by augmenting (enlarging) the jaw, cheeks, and/or chin. Changing facial structures to achieve harmony is achieved through:

- Reduction of facial structures that may include cutting or reducing excess bone and/or soft tissue.
- Augmentation of facial features through the use of implants, bone, cartilage, or soft tissue, to change the proportion and size of the cheeks, chin, nose, and jaw.

How to achieve facial harmony is best evaluated in consultation with a board-certified plastic surgeon or facial plastic surgeon, or in some cases, an oral surgeon. In your consultation, clearly identify the features you wish to change and how you think the change will affect your overall appearance. Also, listen carefully to the surgeon. She or he should recommend a given procedure or procedures and tell you whether or not your goals can realistically be achieved. Write down your questions and the answers. If you don't feel fully confident in both the provider and/or the course of treatment recommended, consult with a second qualified provider.

Achieving facial harmony can be highly gratifying. In cases where very prominent or disfiguring conditions are improved, plastic surgery can truly elevate one's self-confidence and change one's outlook on life. When plastic surgery enhances, corrects, or changes familial traits (features in your appearance that are inherited), family members may sometimes be unsupportive of your desire to alter appearance. If you and your surgeon accept the goals you wish to achieve as realistic and attainable, find someone supportive to help you after surgery. You don't need to be worrying about anyone else while you are recovering.

64. How can the appearance of my nose be improved?

Your nose is an essential organ that allows you to smell, taste, and breathe effectively. It is also the most defining feature of the human face.

Rhinoplasty is surgery of the nose performed to improve appearance and often function. "Rhino" is derived from the Greek term for nose; "plasty" means to form or reshape. Rhinoplasty reshapes the nose to improve appearance and/or breathing.

Are you covered?

Where surgery of the nose is performed to improve breathing function, precertification is required for insurance coverage. Reconstructive nose surgery also may be performed to restore a more normal appearance to a nose that is disfigured due to disease, trauma, or birth defect. Your surgeon's office will assist you by providing the necessary documentation to file with your insurer for authorization prior to surgery. Any reconstructive nose surgery requires careful examination, appropriate documentation, and a defined surgical course in order to obtain insurance coverage.

When rhinoplasty is performed solely to enhance appearance, the procedure is aesthetic and no insurance coverage is available.

In cases where rhinoplasty to improve appearance is performed at the same time as surgery of the nose to improve breathing function, insurance may cover the portion of surgical, anesthesia, and other related fees that apply specifically to the reconstructive portion of the surgery. Precertification is required.

Improving appearance

Nose surgery is the most common facial structural procedure performed to achieve facial harmony. Aesthetic rhinoplasty can accomplish any or all of the following:

- Revision of the nasal bridge—correction of humps or depressions, adjustment of a broad or narrow bridge
- Revision of the nasal tip—reduction of a bulbous tip, changing the angle of the tip or augmenting a poorly projected tip

- Reshaping nostrils, including reduction of enlarged nostrils
- Revision of multiple features of the nose including the size, angles, and curves of the nose in relation and proportion to other facial features

Defining your goals for rhinoplasty may be very simple, or perhaps quite difficult, to express. Communication with your plastic surgeon is key to achieving a good outcome. Be aware, however, that outcomes for rhinoplasty are difficult to fully predict. Bone, cartilage, and soft tissue are confined to a very small space, and tissues all heal differently after surgery. In some cases, more than one procedure may be necessary to achieve your expectations.

Correcting a problem

The most common cause of breathing impairment related to the structure of the nose is a deviated septum. A septum is the main supporting wall of the two sides of the nose. A deviated septum is one that is crooked, dislodged, or displaced. This can result in an obstruction to air as it passes through one or both sides of the nose. Correction requires removal of a portion of the septum and then repositioning. Severe defect in the structure of the septum may require that cartilage or bone be grafted from other areas of the body. Bone or cartilage taken from the back of the ear or from a rib are sometimes used to rebuild the septum and correct other severe nasal deformities. Sometimes, soft tissue grafts and flaps may be used in nasal reconstruction, based on the cause and extent of the deformity. In many cases, reconstruction of severe deformities may require multiple procedures.

According to the American Society of Plastic Surgeons, nose reshaping was the top surgical aesthetic plastic surgery procedure in 2003, with nearly 357,000 procedures performed. In the same survey, nose reshaping was the top aesthetic plastic surgery procedure for men, with nearly 130,000 men having the procedure in 2003.

In 2002, the American Academy of Facial Plastic and Reconstructive Surgeons reported an average of 72 rhinoplasty procedures performed per member, per year, or 6 procedures per month.

Good candidates

Aesthetic rhinoplasty candidates are healthy individuals whose facial growth is completed (generally age 16 and older).

Reconstructive nose surgery may be performed at any age as recommended by a physician. The range is broad: Infants may require reconstruction related to a cleft defect, and elderly patients may undergo reconstruction following tumor removal.

How it's done

Surgery of the nose is generally performed on an outpatient basis, in an office-based, ambulatory-, or hospital-based surgical setting. Anesthesia is usually local anesthesia with intravenous sedation or general anesthesia.

The procedure is generally performed one of two ways:

- A closed procedure, one where incisions are made inside the nose with more limited direct vision and access to the nasal structure.

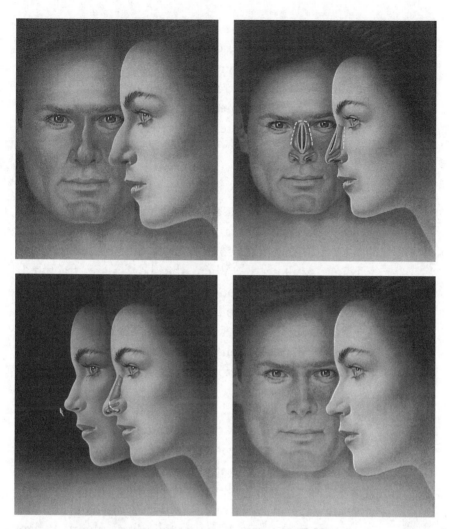

Figure 10 **Rhinoplasty before and after. This is an artist's rendering and does not represent actual patient results. Individual results may vary. Courtesy of the American Society of Plastic Surgeons®. All rights reserved. Learn more at *www.plasticsurgery.org*.**

- An open procedure, where an incision is made at the base of the nose to lift the soft tissue and allow your surgeon direct vision of the underlying structures.

Cartilage and bone may be cut, removed, repositioned, replaced, or grafted to reduce or augment the various structures of your nose. Soft tissue also may be reduced, augmented, or reshaped. Your nose may be "broken" during surgery. This is more correctly defined as an osteotomy, or fracture made in the bones of the nose at a predetermined point. All of the modifications to your nasal structure are precisely planned as part of the course of surgery.

What to expect

Following surgery, nasal packing may be placed to support the structures as they heal. Or, drains may be placed so that fluid comes out of the nose rather than being swallowed. When the bones are fractured, splints may be used outside the nose to further support it during healing. You will look bruised and swollen, particularly in the area underneath the eyes. Additionally, you may find your upper jaw or teeth to be somewhat sore. A soft diet is appropriate for a few days.

Pain is to be expected in the days immediately following surgery. Flexible cold compresses and medication can control and alleviate any swelling and discomfort you experience. It is important that your head is elevated to reduce swelling and bruising and to prevent swallowing of nasal drainage. Nasal discharge will be present in the first 48 hours following surgery. It may be thick and bloody, and moustache dressings will need to be changed frequently to keep you feeling clean and comfortable.

You will likely spend the first day after surgery resting in bed or on the sofa with your head elevated at all times, and you will need to have a responsible adult with you at all times in the first 24 hours following surgery. You will also need to take short walks, with a responsible adult by your side. Do not bend over or lift anything heavy.

Drains are usually removed within a day or two following surgery. Within a week, packing and splints will probably be removed, and swelling and bruising will begin to subside. When you feel ready you can return to normal daily activity, but not vigorous exercise until your surgeon gives you the okay. Do not do any activities that may risk injury to your nose—it can refracture very easily. Within six weeks, most swelling and bruising will no longer be visible, except at the tip. You need to use sun protection for at least the first year following surgery. The structure of your nose and the overlying soft tissues will take at least a year to settle into a final result.

What you need to know

Specific complications following nose surgery include the possibility of bleeding. In addition, infection may develop, and if you have had grafts, they may not take. Excess scar tissue and bony spurs may occur where your nose has been broken. In addition, a broken nose may have bones that dislodge, even if properly supported and protected during healing. As with any surgery that requires anesthesia, there are risks specifically associated with anesthesia.

Nose surgery outcomes are not as predictable as many other surgeries. Although bone and cartilage may be reshaped nicely, that shape may not work well with the soft tissues. The restrictions of your anatomy do not allow for certain changes to be made. For instance, if you have thick skin, you will need much more bone and cartilage to create definition than someone with thin skin. If you have thin skin, every bend in the cartilage will show. Be sure you have thoroughly discussed realistic goals with your surgeon prior to surgery.

Your responsibilities

Smokers will be required to stop smoking for several weeks before surgery, throughout recovery, and for several weeks following surgery. In addition, sun protection and protecting the nose from injury during physical activity are imperative until healing is fully completed, generally for one year.

Your goals

The final results of nose surgery may take a year to fully develop. But even initial results can be very fulfilling to individuals seeking to achieve facial harmony or to correct a prominent or disproportionate nasal feature. The results of rhinoplasty are permanent, although as some individuals age the appearance of the nose may change, including changes in cartilage and a drooping of the nasal tip.

Complements

Aesthetic rhinoplasty may be performed in conjunction with other facial structural procedures, primarily facial implants, to achieve facial harmony. It also may be performed in conjunction with facial rejuvenation procedures to soften the signs of aging.

It's *your* nose. Don't expect that you can bring your surgeon a photo of a nose you like and that rhinoplasty will achieve a similar appearance. It is the composition of all facial features—not just your nose—that together form your appearance. Even if the nose in the photo is closely duplicated in your case, your appearance will not mirror that photo. More often, your nasal structure and soft tissues may not allow for the nose that you think you might like to have; it simply cannot be created. Be sure you have a candid conversation with your surgeon and know what can and cannot be achieved.

If you are considering rhinoplasty and have specific ethnic features, such as Asian, Hispanic, or African American, you should ask any surgeon you consult with about his or her experience in performing rhinoplasty on individuals of similar ethnic origin. Rhinoplasty of the ethnic nose does not mean imposing standards of Caucasian features. Your plastic surgeon should address your individual desires and focus on a more attractive appearance that retains ethnic character, if that is what you want.

65. How can my small chin and jaw, and flat cheeks be improved?

The nose may be the most prominent and central facial feature, but it is the structure of the face as a whole that forms your overall appearance. To achieve facial harmony, facial implants may be helpful to change the size, contours, and angles of the cheek (submalar or malar) region, or the chin and jaw. Implant placement can be performed as a separate procedure or in varying combinations with rhinoplasty or facial rejuvenation surgery.

Facial implants are typically formed of medical-grade solid silicone or other solid substances that can be safely used in the human body. They are specially shaped and sized solid structures that can be

Beauty and Balance

implanted into the face, much like an artificial joint can be implanted in the body with orthopedic surgery.

The key to successful outcomes with facial implants is a careful evaluation of your overall facial structure and appearance: angles, curves, proportions, and prominences. You may be surprised when you consult with a plastic surgeon or facial plastic surgeon about the desire to undergo rhinoplasty and find that, in addition, a chin implant is recommended. Or, you may be considering a face lift for a more youthful appearance and discover that malar or prejowl implants might also be helpful. Your plastic surgeon is listening to your goals, but she or he is also looking for the best possible means to achieve facial harmony. Be certain to have a complete discussion of alternatives and take your time looking in the mirror from all sides. Then make your decision.

Facial implants do not just enhance the size of certain facial features. Some features that are very prominent are brought into proportion when facial implants change the appearance of other facial features—such as using a chin or prejowl implant to bring proportion to a face with a large, broad forehead. Whether facial implants were your initial desire, or suggested by your surgeon, make certain that all aspects and proportions of your face are evaluated before undergoing any procedure to alter your facial structure.

A small or recessed chin is one that in profile does not project evenly or beyond the forehead or mid-face, or that seems to disappear into the neck. Mentoplasty (chin augmentation) with the use of implants can increase the size of the chin, increase how far a chin extends beyond the jaw, or both. Achieving facial harmony and proportion as well as your individual goals for improvement are keys to selecting the right size and shape of an implant for you.

An undefined jaw line is commonly one that disappears into the neck, or one that lacks a definition in angle and proportion from the lower ear to the chin. Without this definition, a person can develop jowls at an early age. Jaw implants are often called prejowl implants because they give increased structure to the area in front of the jowl. (They extend across the chin, along the mandible to the middle of the jaw.) If these implants also have a projection at the chin, they may be called prejowl/chin implants. They are both very helpful in giving balance to a face when the upper two-thirds are proportionately larger than an underdeveloped lower one-third. These implants can improve the hereditary characteristics of a small or weak jaw, or improve appearance as the result of bone loss due to disease or loss of teeth.

A prejowl, prejowl/chin, or chin implant may be placed through an incision inside the mouth between the lower jaw and lower lip, or through an external incision just below and under the chin.

Both the American Society of Plastic Surgeons and the American Academy of Facial Plastic Surgeons reported a significant decrease in chin augmentation over the immediate prior years: ASPS by 39% from 2002 to 2003 and AAFPRS by 29% from 2001 to 2002. In prior years, the number of chin augmentations was relatively stable, nearing 30,000 procedures each year.

If you have a flat, hollow, or undefined mid-face, it can be enhanced through malar or sub-malar augmentation, which are commonly called cheek implants. Cheek implants can be placed high on the cheekbones (malar) or just under the largest projection of the cheeks (sub-malar). These can increase the volume, enhance the curve, and heighten position of the mid-face (malar), or fill a hollow mid-face (submalar). The size and position of cheek implants in relation to your facial structure and goals for harmony are essential to a natural result. Cheek implants that are too large or too low in position can result in an appearance that might well be labeled "chipmunk cheeks." Those that are too high may result in you looking like the Joker character from the Batman comics.

Cheek implants are used to correct features that result from heredity or to improve the signs of aging in the midface, often in conjunction with a face lift. Cheek implants may be placed through incisions inside the lower eyelid, within the hairline at the temples, or though incisions inside the mouth, high in the upper lip.

As recently as 2002, there have been new substances available to slightly increase the volume of the mid-face. The use of some injectable fillers are controversial when used for this purpose and are discussed specifically in Part 11. Injectable fillers are not alternatives to malar implants or a substitute for them. They do not alter the facial structure but only increase the volume of soft tissue. Also, a mid-face lift can fill in malar and submalar tissues that have fallen with age. Again, this procedure provides some soft tissue filling, not a change in the structural support.

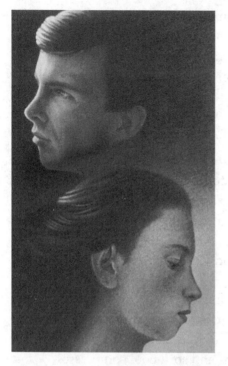 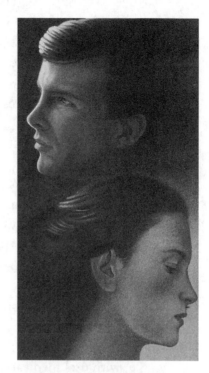

Figure 11   Facial implants before and after. This is an artist's rendering and does not represent actual patient results. Individual results may vary. Courtesy of the American Society of Plastic Surgeons®. All rights reserved. Learn more at *www.plasticsurgery.org*.

Good candidates

Healthy individuals whose facial structural growth has reached maturity, usually after age 16, are good candidates for facial implants.

How it's done

Placement of any solid implant to alter the facial structure requires surgery in an office-based, ambulatory, or hospital operating room setting. Anesthesia ranges from local with oral or intravenous sedation, to general anesthesia depending on the extent of the surgery and your surgeon's recommendations.

Placement of the implants requires a pocket to be formed between the bone and the soft tissues. Internal sutures or medical grade screws may be used to affix the implant in proper position. Incisions will likely be closed with sutures.

What to expect

The structural changes achieved by facial implants are visible immediately following surgery. However, your face will be swollen and bruised. Normal sensation in the area of the implants will be reduced, and your facial movements will be stiff for several days to weeks depending on your individual conditions and treatment.

Soft tissues surrounding the implant may be sore and feel tight as they are stretched over the augmented structures. Pain and discomfort should be controlled with oral medications and soft, cool compresses. A soft or liquid diet may be recommended for the first few days, and you will need to keep your head elevated to reduce any swelling. A responsible adult will need to stay with you at all times for at least 24 hours following surgery. Within a day or two you should be ready for light normal activity.

Some physicians may apply external bandages for a few days following surgery to help support the implant during initial healing; it is important to keep these in place per your surgeon's instructions. Any bandages or stitches will likely be removed within a week following surgery. Swelling and bruising will vastly improve within this period, but significant swelling will remain for several weeks.

Normal activity and fitness can resume within a few weeks of surgery, as long as you don't engage in any activity that could cause injury to your face. In addition, you need to shield the skin surrounding the surgical site from unprotected sun exposure during initial healing as the compromised tissues are susceptible to sunburn and pigment change.

What you need to know

Infection around the implant may require its removal and/or replacement. In addition, if the implant is displaced—if it shifts or moves from its original location—it will require surgical revision. Other complications following surgery include the rare possibility of permanent nerve injury. Deformity of the soft tissues overlying the implant are also possible, but rare. In addition, there are always the risks associated with anesthesia.

Your responsibilities

Following your surgeon's directions is imperative. Infection is more likely if you have incisions inside your mouth. Therefore, even if you are able to brush your teeth comfortably, you should also rinse your mouth with peroxide or an antiseptic solution as recommend by your surgeon. It is especially important to rinse after eating and at bedtime, until the incisions have completely healed.

Smokers will be required to stop smoking for several weeks before surgery and throughout recovery until healing is fully completed.

Your goals

The results of facial implants are visible immediately and may dramatically alter your appearance, or may simply enhance facial harmony. A facial implant can be an immensely gratifying change for individuals with even minor disproportion of facial structures. The facial changes from implants are permanent, although your appearance will naturally continue to change as you age or if you have significant weight change.

The change in you

The structural change after surgery of a disproportionate facial trait will be very obvious to you. But don't be surprised if others can't exactly identify why you look better. They often think it is a weight change or a new hairstyle. Enjoy keeping them guessing.

You may find yourself looking in the mirror often (or multiple mirrors to get a good profile view) as you get used to your new appearance. And you may find that, along with that new appearance, you want to get a new hair style or try new cosmetics. You may find yourself smiling more often. Men who have hidden a small chin behind a beard will likely enjoy a clean-shaven look. All of these things are absolutely normal in accepting your new appearance and the confidence that comes with it.

66. How are protruding or deformed ears corrected?

The Disney story about the baby elephant Dumbo teaches us that we all are special, based on those things that make us unique as individuals. But there is nothing special about a child who is ridiculed or teased about having "Dumbo ears." Dumbo may have used his ears to fly and to win back the approval of the circus ringmaster, but there is little a child can do make his or her prominent ears a magical asset.

There was a time when surgery to correct prominent or "Dumbo" ears (called otoplasty) was referred to as "pinning back." Today, a pinned look is not considered a desirable outcome of surgery of the ear or otoplasty. Otoplasty can improve the aesthetic appearance of protruding ears to create a more natural contour and softer appearance.

Although otoplasty is more often performed on children, adults frequently undergo the procedure to improve appearance that may have bothered them since childhood. Many of these adults have had hairstyles that covered their ears for most of their lives.

A new angle

Ears that protrude are sometimes called "Dumbo" ears, but, in fact, it is rare that ears are overly large in size. More often, prominent ears protrude from the head due to deeply cupped cartilage and/or a lack of normal folding of the cartilage inside the upper portion of the ear. Protruding ears can make a child the subject of teasing and ridicule by peers. This can significantly affect self-esteem at a very early and influential age when self-confidence is critical to a child's social development and emotional health.

In the past, protruding ears were often corrected by removing a piece of cartilage from the back of the ear, then pulling the ear closer to the head by closing the incision. This technique caused a very unnatural appearance, as it distorted and sharpened the natural folds in the ear. Today, similar techniques are used; however, the incision patterns are designed to maintain or create natural curves in the ear as well as improve the angle of the ear with respect to the head. The ear

Beauty and Balance

may actually be weakened and folded back onto itself to achieve a natural outcome. Sometimes cartilage may be removed from the cupped portion inside the ear (called the "concha") when this area is overly deep. Other, more rare ear deformities that may be treated with reconstructive plastic surgery include:

- A lop, cup, or constricted ear that may protrude, may be small in overall size and circumference, and may be folded, or may have a flattened rim or folds. In some cases the ear may be in a lower than normal position on the head. This can occur on one or both sides (that is, unilaterally or bi-laterally) and may or may not affect hearing.
- Stahl's ear is distorted in shape and may have a "Dr. Spock" like appearance. The condition generally does not impair hearing.
- A hidden ear, called cryptotia, is one that appears buried into the skull, when in fact a portion of the ear is folded into and buried underneath the scalp.
- Microtia is a severe ear deformity where the ear formation is incomplete. The ear may have few if any protruding or normal folds and components of the ear structure. Hearing may be impaired or lost as the ear may be missing the external auditory or hearing canal. Reconstruction of microtia requires staged surgical procedures to create a more normal external ear.

Reconstructive procedures in any of these cases require a highly individualized approach, and in some cases includes a team: surgeon, pediatrician, speech pathologist, auditory specialist, and a social worker. Reconstruction may occur with many stages. Therefore, you must first consult with a board-certified plastic surgeon or facial plastic surgeon experienced with ear surgery. That surgeon should define the course of surgery and treatment recommended, and recommend or pull together a team of specialists.

How it's done

In children, ear surgery will usually be performed using general anesthesia; in adults, general anesthesia or local anesthesia with oral or IV sedation may be used. Surgery will be performed in an operating room that is office-based, in an ambulatory surgical facility, or in a hospital setting.

Surgery to improve protruding ears, with or without excision of cartilage, will require sutures to form the new shape of the ear and hold the ear position in place as it heals. Surgery may be performed on both ears even though only one appears to protrude. This will achieve the most uniform result. This type of ear surgery can be performed on an outpatient basis.

Reconstruction may require grafting of cartilage taken from other areas of the body, such as the rib, or a piece of bone from the base of the skull or the hip. In some cases, synthetic substances may be an alternative to grafts taken from a patient's own body. Complete lack of an outer ear due to congenital deformity or loss from disease or planned or accidental amputation may be treated with an implant. Surgical implantation of prosthetics today are very natural in appearance and to the touch. The duration of reconstruction or number of procedures required to achieve final outcomes can only be defined on a case-by-case basis. Make certain your surgeon defines each phase of the surgical plan for you or your child. Most cases can be performed on an outpatient basis.

Good candidates

Surgery to correct protruding ears can be performed as early as age 4 or when the ears have fully grown, around the age of 6 or 7. It is best to plan surgery when and if the child shows a desire to have the condition corrected and is able to communicate that desire. In addition, a child must be able to understand what the surgical experience includes, as well as be cooperative post-operatively. He or she must accept patient responsibilities such as wearing bandages or dressings during healing. Adults can also find ear surgery to be fulfilling and are equally good candidates if they are healthy.

Reconstructive surgery to correct deformities or absence of the ear can be performed at any age.

What to expect

Bandages will conceal the new position or shape of the reconstructed ear or repositioned ear. They are essential to support and protect the ear during initial phases of healing, and in some cases they actually help to mold the skin to the newly shaped underlying cartilage. There may be a throbbing or dull pain that is easily controlled by oral medications. In most cases, light normal activity can be resumed as soon as the patient feels ready, which may be within a day or less following surgery.

Headache and discomfort may persist for a few days. Sites from which grafts have been taken will be sore and may be red, swollen, or slightly bruised.

Within a week your surgeon will remove any bandages or dressings to reveal the new shape of the ear. Any stitches that require removal will likely be removed at the same time, or within a few days.

Normal activity can resume as soon as a patient feels ready, or when your surgeon allows. Most children can resume active play as soon they are ready as long as the ears and graft sites are protected from injury. In some cases your surgeon may suggest a protective headband to be worn daily or only at night to help maintain the new position of the ear.

What you need to know

Pooling of blood underneath the skin at the surgical site may occur. If there is a significant amount, it will have to be drained, otherwise the underlying cartilage can warp and result in a deformity of the cartilage often called "cauliflower ear." Infection is also a very rare possibility. This must be treated aggressively, because cartilage has a poor blood supply and doesn't respond well to antibiotics alone. As with any surgery, there are risks associated with anesthesia.

Additional risks in outcome include the possibility of overcorrection or under-correction of protrusion. Because cartilage is soft and flexible, the way it reacts to reshaping may not be fully predictable. Slight asymmetry of the ears is also possible, but some mild asymmetry is normal and not often noticeable.

Your responsibilities

Whether you are an adult or child, it is imperative to follow all of your surgeon's instructions, including keeping any bandages or dressings intact. Although the dressings can feel cumbersome and itchy, it is vital that they not be removed, displaced, or dislodged in any way until your surgeon removes them. The dressings are important to allow the skin to mold to the cartilage and prevent blood from pooling. Sun protection is important postoperatively to prevent permanent discoloration of the ears.

Adult patients who smoke will be required to stop smoking for several weeks before surgery and for several weeks during recovery.

Your goals

The results of ear surgery are permanent. Otoplasty results are visible as soon as bandages are removed, although there will be visible swelling and bruising. Reconstruction will be visible over time as various stages of the course of treatment are completed.

More than just appearances

Ear surgery, when performed by appropriately credentialed and experienced plastic or facial plastic surgeons, has a high record of safety and satisfaction. Children who undergo the procedure may gain vastly elevated self-esteem. They may show improvement in school and social skills, or may experience a much happier daily life when they are no longer subjected to ridicule by their peers.

67. Are there other plastic surgery procedures of the facial structures?

There are two very specialized segments of plastic surgery that relate to reconstructive surgery of the facial structures. Craniofacial surgery is specific to the structures of the cranium (head and face), and maxillofacial surgery is specific to the region of the mandible (lower jaw) and maxilla (upper jaw). Craniofacial surgery is a subspecialty of plastic surgery that should be performed by a board-certified plastic or facial plastic surgeon with added training and experience in this very specialized field. Maxillofacial procedures may similarly be performed by these surgeons and also by board-certified oral surgeons with specific training in maxillofacial surgery.

The American Society for Maxillofacial Surgery represents maxillofacial and craniofacial surgeons in the United States who specialize in bone and soft tissue reconstruction and enhancement of the face. *www.maxface.org*

According to the American Society of Plastic Surgeons, just over 90,000 reconstructive maxillofacial procedures were performed in 2003 by their members. This number does not include tumor removal or correction of birth defects.

PART TEN

Looking Younger: Surgical Facial Rejuvenation

Can plastic surgery reverse signs of aging?

What are blepharoplasty, brow lift, and rhytidectomy procedures?

When is a limited facelift appropriate?

What are the alternatives to surgical rejuvenation?

More ...

Who doesn't want to look young? Or look as young as you feel? Or maybe look your age? Or not look like you are aging? In our society, youth, beauty, and vitality are often viewed as far more preferable than naturally aging. Humans have always sought out ways to look and feel younger. Medicine can improve our health and prolong our lives. But the one thing we cannot prevent is the process of aging.

Plastic surgery can, however, slow the changes aging produces in our appearance. Facial rejuvenation surgery is one of the most rapidly growing categories in plastic surgery both in the number of procedures performed each year and in an expanding age range among patients. It is second only to the nonsurgical means of improving (rejuvenating) an aging appearance.

68. What is surgical rejuvenation of the face?

Surgical rejuvenation of the face includes procedures that essentially restore a more youthful appearance to an individual. These surgical procedures are designed to make you look like a more youthful version of yourself. People from many income levels and of many age groups (even as young as their thirties) are undergoing surgical rejuvenation. Not all of these patients are women, either.

We all develop the signs of aging a little differently, and the signs appear at different times in our lives. But aging is not only a result of time—heredity and environment have their influences, too. Rejuvenative procedures target the specific signs of aging in all areas of the face and neck. These can be performed individually, or multiple procedures can be performed in one or more surgical sessions. The procedures include:

- Eyelid surgery: to restore a smooth contour to the upper eyelid, and/or correct bagging of the lower eyelid.
- Brow lift: to raise a drooping brow and/or smooth furrows in the forehead region.
- Face lift: to restore and smooth contours to the midface, jowls, and neck
- Autologous enhancement: using your own tissue to augment facial areas
- Non-autologous enhancement: using tissue or implants from other sources to augment facial areas

Appropriate providers of rejuvenative plastic surgery procedures of the face include plastic surgeons certified by the American Board of Plastic Surgery and board-certified facial plastic surgeons. In addition, board-certified ophthalmologists with added training in ophthalmic plastic surgery (or occuloplastic surgery) are appropriate providers of rejuvenative procedures of the eyes and surrounding tissues.

There are also nonsurgical means to soften the signs of aging or improve an aging appearance. These are more commonly called minimally invasive therapies and are addressed specifically in Part 11.

69. Can I stop my face and body from aging?

Rejuvenation procedures can return your appearance to a more youthful one, but they do not stop the aging process. Nothing can stop aging completely. We can, however, help to slow some of the problems of aging through healthy lifestyles. By seeing our doctors regularly, eating the right foods, and exercising, we can take some control over our health. Good skin care and protection from the sun are also important parts of that control. While human growth hormones (HGH), phyto-esters (plant compounds), vitamins, and herbs are continuously researched, it is not yet proven whether they are effective or, in some cases, even safe.

There are two factors that speed up the process of facial aging:

- Environmental influences, such as sun exposure, pollution, and dryness
- Poor health, smoking, weight changes, and stress

You cannot prevent normal aging of your face and body. But you can focus on a healthy lifestyle to minimize further damage. And, if you don't want to accept the signs of aging when they appear, you might consider surgical rejuvenation.

70. How can baggy eyelids be corrected?

The eyelid area is one of the first regions of the face to show the signs of aging. The skin of the eyelids is the thinnest and most delicate in the entire body. At the same time, the eyelid area is one of the most animated parts of the face, with strong muscles creating multiple expressions. It is, therefore, understandable why eyelid surgery is one of the most popular rejuvenative plastic surgery procedures. Additionally, inherited features such as shallow bone structure and a down-turn of the outer corner of the eye tend to cause bagging of the lower eyelid at a much earlier age.

The appearance of saggy eyelids at any age can make a well-rested person look tired and a happy person look sad or even angry. Eyelid surgery (called blepharoplasty) improves the appearance of the upper and/or lower eyelids by restoring or creating a smooth upper eyelid contour and correcting excess drooping or puffiness (bags) in the lower eyelid. Eyelid surgery does not change the position or nature of the eyebrows. (The procedure to correct these conditions is a brow lift.) In addition, eyelid surgery does not correct crow's feet, although it may improve them somewhat. Canthopexy and canthoplasty are related procedures that tighten the outer tendons in the lower eyelid to uplift the outer corner and prevent drooping.

Eyelid surgery may be performed by a board-certified plastic surgeon, a board certified ophthalmologist with added surgical training in occuloplastic or ophthalmic plastic surgery, or a facial plastic surgeon (an otolaryngologist with added training in facial plastic surgery).

Are you covered?

Eyelid surgery is generally an aesthetic procedure and is not eligible for reimbursement by insurers. Occasionally, when the upper eyelids are so lax that vision is obscured, insurance may cover a portion of the procedure. A thorough eye exam, including visual fields, must be performed by your ophthalmologist, and pre-certification must be obtained.

Good candidates

Good candidates for eyelid surgery include healthy adult men and women with puffy or sagging eyelids. There are certain conditions that require special con-

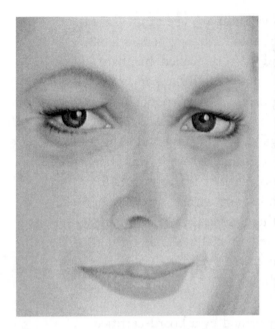
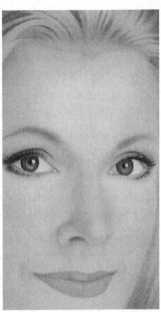

Figure 12   Eyelid surgery (blepharoplasty). This is an artist's rendering and does not represent actual patient results. Individual results may vary. Courtesy of the American Society of Plastic Surgeons®. All rights reserved. Learn more at *www.plasticsurgery.org.*

siderations before eyelid surgery. If you have eye diseases such as glaucoma, detached retina, Grave's disease, or other diseases that affect your vision, you should have the approval of your ophthalmologist prior to surgery. You should also have approval by your primary care physician if you have systemic diseases such as thyroid disease, high blood pressure, bleeding disorders, or diabetes.

How it's done

Eyelid surgery can be performed on the upper eyelid, the lower eyelid, or both.

Upper eyelids

Upper eyelid surgery restores a smoother and more alert appearance to the upper eyelid. It requires an incision generally made in or below the natural crease of the upper eyelid, through which:

- Excess skin and tissue is excised (cut out)
- Fat may be removed or redistributed
- The muscles of the eyelid may be repositioned or a portion may be removed

The length and shape of the incisions depend on the degree of excess skin that exists. The incision is closed with removable or absorbable very fine stitches.

Lower eyelids

For lower eyelids, the puffiness and bagginess of the lower eyelid that creates a tired or sad appearance can be corrected three ways:

- Through an incision hidden inside the lower eyelid (for fat removal)
- Through an external incision just below the lower eyelashes (for skin and/or fat removal)
- Through an incision in the upper eyelid (for horizontal tightening and/or an upward slope)

Fat is removed through an internal or external incision. Only external incisions allow for removal of excess skin. When the lower lid is lax or severely sagging, canthoplasty or canthopexy can be performed. These procedures tighten the lower lid in its horizontal dimension and may upturn the outer corner to varying degrees. The lower lid outer attachments to

Looking Younger: Surgical Facial Rejuvenation

the bone (tendons) are changed in order to correct the lax eyelid. Canthoplasty repositions and reinforces the lower eyelid by cutting and permanently repositioning the lower eyelid tendons. Canthopexy stabilizes and may upturn the lower eyelid tendons using an internal suture to anchor the tendon to bone. Incisions are closed with fine sutures.

What to expect

When performed alone, eyelid surgery may be performed under local anesthesia, often with sedation, or under general anesthesia. Eyelid surgery is an outpatient procedure in most cases, performed in an office-based, ambulatory-, or hospital-based surgical facility.

When your procedure is completed, your eyes will likely be teary, with somewhat blurry vision. Ointment may be applied to your eyes. Your eyes may be very puffy, swollen, and begin to bruise. You will be released to the care of a responsible adult family member, friend, or caregiver who will need to stay with and assist you for at least the first 24 hours following surgery. Cool compresses will help to alleviate any discomfort as will oral medications. It is imperative that you rest and sleep in an elevated position and that you not bend forward for any reason.

You will not be able to wear contact lenses until your surgeon advises that you may resume doing so. If you wear hard lenses, you may need refitting. To keep your eyes well lubricated, you will be given special drops to use as directed, and you will also be given instructions for cleansing your incisions and ointment to help them heal.

You may resume light daily activity as soon as you feel ready. You must not, however, do any bending or heavy lifting. You will likely be sensitive to bright light, and your eyes will feel dry for a while. Be sure to use your drops and ointment, as prescribed, to alleviate dry eye conditions.

What you need to know

The risks and complications of eyelid surgery include bleeding, prolonged bruising, poor healing at the incision site, injury to the surface of the eye such as corneal abrasion, and dry eye. Your eyes will feel somewhat tight and dry for the first few months following surgery; this is not a complication. Continued difficulty in fully closing your eyes is possible, but rare. With lower eyelid surgery there is the added risk of a pulling down of the lower eyelid. Blindness has been reported after fat removal due to bleeding behind the eye. This is a very, very rare complication. Permanent dry eye is also possible, especially in patients who have some dryness preoperatively. It is a good idea to check your tear production prior to surgery so that your plastic surgeon can plan accordingly. The other complications are generally correctable when eyelid surgery is performed by an experienced, and appropriately qualified, surgeon. In addition, there are risks associated with anesthesia.

Your responsibilities

Patients will be advised to stop smoking for several weeks before eyelid surgery and until healing is complete. In addition, you will likely be advised to stop taking certain medications and supplements for several days prior to surgery and immediately afterward. The success of your surgery is greatly influenced by wound care taken and the use of prescribed eyedrops and ointments.

Your goals

Correction of the upper eyelid and the smoother contour of the lower eyelid will be obscured by swelling and bruising immediately following surgery. These changes should subside greatly within the first week and continue to improve over the next two to four months. Soon after sutures are removed and incisions have healed, you may use makeup to camouflage bruising and scars. The scars from your external incisions will continue to change and fade over the next six months or more. Over time, you may not even notice these scars; they are placed so that they are concealed in the natural crease of the upper eyelid and by the lower lash line. All scars are, however, permanent.

Your view

To friends and family you will look well-rested and happier. Some may not even relate this to an improvement in the appearance of your eyes. They will often think you have been on a very relaxing vacation, or that the stress and strain of daily life have lessened.

Eyelid surgery is among the top five aesthetic plastic surgery procedures for both men and women, according to data in 2003 from both the American Society of Plastic Surgeons and the American Society for Aesthetic Plastic Surgery. It is the most commonly performed surgical rejuvenation procedure. ASPS reports nearly 247,000 procedures performed in 2003. According to the American Academy of Facial Plastic Surgeons, in 2002, blepharoplasty was the most commonly performed aesthetic procedure among their members.

71. Can a hooded or furrowed brow be corrected?

A brow lift is surgery to improve or reposition a low, hooded brow, as well as vertical "frown lines" that develop above the bridge of the nose, between the eyes. A sagging, furrowed forehead and brow that develop with age can make a content individual appear angry or scowling, and a well-rested individual appear tired and drawn. Brow lift restores a more youthful and alert appearance to the brow region.

Often, people ask for eyelid surgery when a brow lift more accurately corrects their conditions. Raising a drooping brow can somewhat improve the appearance of the upper eyelid. But brow lift alone does nothing to change the contour of the upper eyelid and eyelid surgery does not raise a drooping brow. Frequently, both procedures are performed together to create a soft, well-rested appearance to the upper eyelid and brow.

Brow lift is most often performed by a board-certified plastic surgeon or board-certified otolaryngologist with a certificate of added qualification in facial plastic surgery.

Are you covered?

Brow lift is an aesthetic procedure and not eligible for insurance reimbursement. Rarely, if a brow is deformed due to previous trauma to the brow nerves, insurance may cover the procedure. Precertification is always necessary.

Good candidates

Good candidates for brow lift are men and women who do not have serious health conditions. Contrary to what some may believe, even men with significant hair loss can be brow lift candidates.

How it's done

Brow lift may be performed several ways. The technique that is right for you is determined by your appearance and anatomy, your goals for a brow lift, and the degree of correction necessary to achieve those goals.

The endoscopic technique is somewhat similar to some orthopaedic joint surgeries or other limited incision surgeries that use a surgical telescope. With this technique, multiple limited incisions are made within or at the hairline. Special instruments are used to pull the deep tissues upward and the muscles that cause vertical creases are separated.

A brow lift may also be performed using incisions:

- Across the top of the head within the hairline (called a coronal incision)
- At the front of the hairline
- Through the upper eyelid

A coronal incision allows for removal of excess skin, if necessary. The incision at the front of the hairline may be combined with the endoscopic lift in patients with a very high forehead. The upper eyelid incision involves cutting those muscles that pull the brows downward. With any technique, the muscles that allow you to make expressions that furrow or crease your brow can be separated so that you cannot make these expressions in the future. Where muscle and other tissues are repositioned, external and/or internal sutures, screws, or other fixating devices may be used to hold the tissues in place. Removable stitches or special metal clips will be used to close your incisions.

What to expect

Brow lift can be performed under local anesthesia with intravenous sedation, or general anesthesia. The procedure is performed on an outpatient basis, in your surgeon's office-, ambulatory-, or hospital-based surgical facility.

When your procedure is completed you will likely feel a dull headache, soreness at the incision sites, and some swelling. Your head may be tightly wrapped and you may have a small thin tube placed to drain any excess fluid. You will be released to the care of a responsible adult friend, family member, or caregiver who must stay with you for at least 24 hours following your surgery. You will be told not to bend down or do any heavy lifting. And, you will need to sleep and rest in an elevated position. There will be swelling and bruising during the first several days following surgery. Oral medication and soft cool compresses should control any discomfort you may experience.

You will be able to shower and wash your hair when drains and dressings are removed and your plastic surgeons gives you permission to do so. Stitches or staples to close your incisions will be removed within one to two weeks; if external screws were used, these may remain in place a little longer. You will be ready for more normal daily activity within two to three weeks.

What you need to know

The risks and complications of brow lift surgery include hematoma (collection of blood beneath the skin) and poor healing. Hair loss at the incision sites may occur, especially with a coronal incision. In addition, you will have numbness within the scalp that is usually temporary. This is due to swelling around the sensory nerves. In very rare cases, you may experience brow paralysis that may or may not resolve. Facial asymmetry (one brow higher than the other) may occur, although this may very well have been the case prior to surgery and now is simply more visible. The brows may initially appear high, but they will relax to a more normal position as swelling diminishes.

Although not a complication, one of the less desirable outcomes of a brow lift using a coronal incision is that you will likely have an elevated hairline. For any individual who already has a high hairline this can be especially disconcerting. Therefore, it is best to thoroughly discuss all of your options and the associated outcomes with your surgeon prior to surgical brow lift. (You may need an incision in the front of your hairline to give you a lower forehead.)

Your responsibilities

Smokers will be required to stop smoking prior to surgery and during recovery. As well, you will be required to stop taking certain medications, vitamins, or supplements prior to surgery and during immediate recovery. You must follow all of your surgeon's instructions for wound cleansing and for wearing dressings or head garments.

Looking Younger: Surgical Facial Rejuvenation

Your goals, your experience

Within two to four weeks you will see most swelling diminish and will be able to do regular daily activity and exercise. It will take months for all swelling to diminish. The results, although permanent, will change as your face continues to age. However, without the ability to create certain expressions the likelihood of forming deep furrows and creases is greatly diminished, and the smoothness of the brow will bring you back many years.

The rejuvenating benefits of brow lift surgery should help you to appear happier, more youthful, and well rested. In the first few days following surgery, you may not feel happy or well rested. But within a few weeks the outcomes will be apparent. Others will most likely not realize that the changes are from plastic surgery.

Of special note: Your surgeon may recommend Botox® Cosmetic therapy injections prior to your procedure to relax the muscles that will be repositioned or following surgery to help maintain the results of brow lift over a longer period of time. Read all the questions in Chapter 11 on Botox® therapy if you are considering a brow lift.

According to the American Society of Plastic Surgeons, brow lift procedures decreased in number from 2000 to 2003 by 52% percent, or from nearly 121,000 procedures to just under 58,000. Why the sharp drop? Likely it is the rise of Botox® as an alternative, non-invasive treatment that provides a temporary, excellent, and safe means to soften brow furrows and creases. Botox does not, however, achieve the same long-lasting results of a surgical brow lift.

72. How is an aging face or neck improved?

A facelift (rhytidectomy) is rejuvenative plastic surgery of the mid-face region, the lower face, including the jowls, and the neck. Rhytidectomy lifts and smoothes the skin of the face and neck. A superficial musculoaponeurotic system (SMAS) procedure "lifts" or repositions the underlying facial muscles as well as the skin. The SMAS facelift was developed in the 1970s in Europe and quickly popularized in the United States. A rhytidectomy and SMAS correct the conditions that contribute to an aging appearance. These conditions are caused by:

- Sagging facial and neck muscles
- Decrease in and downward displacement of facial fat
- Sagging lax skin of the face and neck

Specifically, a facelift softens and improves:

- Saggy, loose jowls that may result in a poorly defined jaw line or one that disappears into the neck
- A sagging neck that may appear as a double chin
- Vertical banding or chords that develop in the neck (platysmal bands)
- Nasolabial folds (the crease that extend from the corners of the nose to the mouth)
- Marionette lines, those creases from the outer corner of the mouth to the chin

Although the nasolabial folds and marionette lines are improved, they will not disappear. In some cases, improvement in the neck may also require a platysmaplasty, which is a procedure to tie the vertical muscle bands together under the chin.

A facelift restores a softer, smoother, more youthful appearance. Following a facelift you should appear more rested, uplifted, and happy as opposed to looking tight or "done." You also will look like a much younger version of yourself. Appropriate providers of the facelift procedure are board-certified plastic surgeons and facial plastic surgeons.

Are you covered?

Facelift is an aesthetic procedure and is not eligible for insurance coverage. There may be exceptions where conditions such as Bell's palsy or stroke have resulted in paralysis and created severe asymmetry in the face. However, even with these conditions, coverage is rare and requires precertification.

Good candidates

Good candidates for facelift are men and women of any age who are in good overall health and wish to restore a more youthful appearance that reflects the vitality they

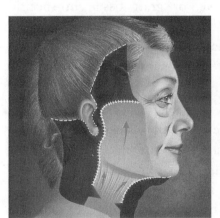 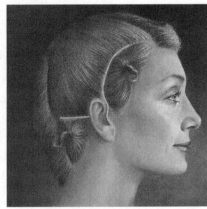

Figure 13   Facelift (rhytidectomy). This is an artist's rendering and does not represent actual patient results. Individual results may vary. Courtesy of the American Society of Plastic Surgeons®. All rights reserved. Learn more at *www.plasticsurgery.org*.

feel. In addition, good candidates are individuals without chronic diseases that may impair healing or that may be life-threatening. Your plastic surgeon should be in close communication with your primary care physician if you have any serious medical condition.

How it's done

A rhytidectomy begins with a continuous incision on each side of the face. The incisions begin in the temples just behind or at the hairline, continue downward into the natural curve of the ear, go around the earlobe and extend upward behind the ear and back into the hairline. Differences in the procedure will be based on the specific areas to be addressed in your case and your plastic surgeon's preferences. Through the incisions your plastic surgeon may:

- Elevate the skin as a flap
- Reposition and tighten or suspend the facial soft tissues in a SMAS surgery (deep plane and/or even deeper plane over the bone)
- Redistribute, remove, or graft tissue in specific areas of the face
- Repair the platysmal bands of the neck
- Redrape the skin, removing any excess

The result of these components of a facelift is a restoration, to a more youthful position, of the internal soft tissues of the face and neck as well as a redraping of the skin with removal of the excess. The hairline should also be treated to bring it to a natural level. Incisions will vary somewhat depending on the amount of skin removed, the direction of skin pull, and the preference of your surgeon. Additional incisions may be made around the sideburns and at the hairline behind the ear to bring the hair closer to the ear.

The incisions will then be closed with stitches and possible staples in the scalp. Drains or internal glue may be used. An additional incision may be required just below the chin to better treat conditions of the neck and remove excess fat deposits in the neck. Liposuction techniques may also be used to reduce fat in the neck, jowls, and some areas of the face.

To achieve facial harmony, discussed in Part 9, a facelift with a deeper plane treatment and/or plastysmaplasty may be combined with brow and eyelid surgery. The use of facial implants to alter the structure of the face may also be recommended in conjunction with a facelift. Depending upon the condition of your face and neck at the time of consultation, combined procedures are frequently recommended so that different parts of your face balance well. Facial harmony is very important if you want to achieve a natural postoperative appearance. While your plastic surgeon is listening to your goals for surgery, she or he should also be taking into consideration achieving facial harmony in any course of treatment recommended.

What to expect

A facelift is usually performed under general anesthesia or local anesthesia with sedation in your plastic surgeon's office-based surgical facility, or in an ambulatory- or hospital-based surgical setting. Depending on your medical condition and length of surgery, it may be performed on an outpatient basis. An overnight hospital stay or recovery in a special postoperative facility may be recommended.

When your surgery is completed, your head will likely be wrapped in bandages; some surgeons may use elastic bandages or special compression wraps. You will feel soreness and some numbness in the face. You may have a small flexible tube placed in your incisions for a few days to drain any excess fluid that accumulates. You will be swollen and bruised. All of these conditions are to be expected, and discomfort can be controlled with oral medications and cool compresses that are soft and flexible.

If your procedure is performed on an outpatient basis, you will be released to a responsible adult family member, friend, or caregiver who must remain with you to assist you for at least 24 hours following surgery. It may be uncomfortable to open your mouth, speak, or eat. A soft diet may be appropriate for a few days. You will be told not to bend down or lower your head for any reason. When resting and sleeping you must remain in an elevated position. This is essential to reduce swelling or bleeding and to allow excess fluid to drain. Light daily activity can resume as soon as you feel ready, but you will likely spend the first few days in simple, quiet activities such as reading or watching television.

Within one to two weeks, your condition will begin to improve rapidly. Stitches will be removed and you will be able to resume more normal activity. You should be able to camouflage bruising with cosmetics at this time, as long as your plastic surgeon says this is okay. It usually takes two to three weeks before you will want to be seen in public.

What you need to know

Surgical facelift is a safe procedure with good outcomes when performed by properly trained and skilled plastic surgeons. Risks associated with a rhytidectomy include bleeding beneath the skin, asymmetry (where both sides do not appear the same), hair loss at the incision sites, and thickening of scars. You will experience numbness for several months in the cheeks; this is not a complication. Although rare, nerve injury may occur, leading to weakness of a portion of the face for several months, or even permanently. You may need minor revisions to achieve your goals when tissues begin to loosen. There are also the associated risks of anesthesia.

Your responsibilities

Smoking can significantly impair healing and the opportunity for good outcomes. Smokers must refrain from smoking for several weeks before surgery and throughout the complete recovery period. In addition, following all of your surgeon's directions is imperative to improve your chances of a good outcome.

Your goals

It may take as many as four to six weeks before most swelling and bruising subsides and your skin returns to a more normal hue. During this time, you may wish to choose a hairstyle that lightly covers the area in front of your ears while the scars from your incisions continue to improve. These scars are permanent, but rarely visible after several months, if placed well.

Sun protection is essential not only in the early stages of healing, but for life. Exposure to ultraviolet rays is a leading factor contributing to the breakdown of facial elastic tissues contributing to aging of the face. Your face will continue to age naturally, but you will be continuing this process from a much younger point.

Your lift

Today, the techniques used in facelift procedures should not produce the tight, unnatural, and wind-swept appearance associated with facelifts of the past. The results are a natural restoration of your more youthful self. A facelift can lift your spirits and confidence, too. To look as youthful and vibrant as you feel is immensely satisfying to many men and women. Other people may not realize the cause of your more youthful appearance. They often think you had a restful vacation or that your hairstylist has done wonders.

According the American Society of Plastic Surgeons, nearly 129,000 facelifts were performed in 2003.

Note: Botox® Cosmetic therapy has been used and is recommended by some plastic surgeons to relax the platysmal bands in the neck prior to facelift, thereby improving surgical outcomes.

73. What if I don't want or need a full facelift?

The first innovation in surgical rejuvenation procedures to really change the facelift was the SMAS, introduced in the 1970s (see Question 72). Over the next few decades it has evolved to be the standard technique in facelifting. The next innovation to facelift surgery was introduced in the early 1990s and has only recently become more mainstream. Pioneers in plastic surgery introduced less invasive forms of the facelift, specifically to address the face that is showing the signs of age in only limited areas, not necessarily all over.

At present, there are multiple techniques and names for these less invasive and more limited forms of a facelift. A "midfacelift" is a term commonly used in media to describe the limited procedure that addresses the cheek area. Others have been referred to as "ponytail friendly" procedures, because the incision pattern of a full facelift is not made. It is more appropriate, however, to call any one of these procedures a limited-incision facelift. An S-lift (the name derived from the short S-shaped incision made in the hairline below the temples) is another name commonly used for a limited incision facelift as is the term endoscopically assisted facelift. Although the mid face is most often the area treated, some procedures correct only the jowls and others only the neck.

These procedures are not a substitute for a full facelift. Although they sound less serious than a facelift, they are, nonetheless, surgical procedures that can change the anatomy of your face. Don't be swayed by fancy marketing such as "incisionless" facelift or "lunchtime" facelift. They are surgical procedures that require incisions, anesthesia, and recovery time. They also have potential complications, as do all surgical procedures. Furthermore, the results may not last long, and it may be more difficult to perform a full facelift at a later date.

"Limited incision" facelifts are also limited facelifts. Good candidates for these more limited procedures are younger individuals with aging isolated to the mid face or jowl. In these patients, excess skin is not the problem. The offending aging features may be:

• An exaggerated tear trough (hollowing below the eye)

- Flattening of the cheeks or downward migration of underlying soft tissue
- Prominent nasolaial folds (those from the nose to the mouth)
- Early marionette lines (from the outer corner of the mouth to the chin).

Many of the same techniques performed in a full facelift are performed in a limited fashion to improve these conditions, often through smaller incisions and in some cases with the assistance of endoscopic techniques (the use of a surgical telescope). Limited facelift procedures are highly individualized based on your anatomy and your surgeon's preference and experience.

The procedures use variations of facelift incision patterns and/or may include incisions in the lower eyelid or high inside the upper lip. Through these incisions your plastic surgeon will address the conditions that have been defined in your consultation. Read all of the information on a facelift carefully. Your experience may be the same as a full facelift, or your recovery may be shorter. Your experience is fully dependent on the techniques used, areas to be treated, and degree of correction.

While a limited incision facelift is not an uncommon procedure, it is still relatively new in the scope of plastic surgery. Very different and often innovative techniques are used. Therefore, only a board-certified plastic or facial plastic surgeon experienced in these techniques as well as full facelifts should be consulted.

Are you covered?

A limited incision or endoscopic facelift is purely aesthetic and not eligible for any insurance coverage.

What you need to know

You need to know the possible risks and complications of a full facelift, as they *all* apply with limited techniques as well. You may initially appear over-lifted and it may take as much as six months or more for your true results to appear. As you continue to age, these areas may remain high while other areas of the face and neck sag. You may then need a full facelift to achieve facial harmony.

Your goals

If your goals are to correct specific aspects of facial aging or to delay the need for a full facelift, then limited techniques may be right for you. The results of a facelift with limited incision techniques are permanent, but your face will continue to age. Consider these procedures an intermediate step to delay the need for a full facelift and to restore a youthful appearance by correcting the signs of aging as they appear.

There are no data yet reported on limited incision facelift techniques alone, but the gaining popularity is clearly attributed to the fact that in 2003 issue of *Vogue* carried three articles that touched on the subject, with additional media coverage in magazines, newspapers, and television.

74. How is a double chin or droopy neck corrected?

An article published in 2003 in the American women's magazine, *Vogue*, stated that at age 40, a woman's neck disappears. Although this statement is a gross exaggeration, it is true that tissues do start to fall, obscuring the jowl-to-neck demarcation.

The aging neck is best treated by full facelift and SMAS surgery, with or without platysmaplasty. Other means of treatment include:

• Varying degrees of limited incision facelift to correct mildly sagging skin and to remove or reposition fat in the neck
• Platysmaplasty alone to correct banding or vertical cords in the neck
• Liposuction alone to remove excess fat that has deposited under the chin and improve the neck contour

Most commonly, these procedures are recommended for younger patients where excess skin is minimal and not the primary factor in the aged appearance of the neck. Sometimes these procedures are labeled a "neck lift," but in fact, lifting the neck is part of a facelift.

Your goals, your plan

If your goals for plastic surgery are to improve the aging appearance of your neck, your plan should include consulting with a board-certified plastic surgeon or facial plastic surgeon. The recommendation of procedures or techniques to best achieve your goals should only be defined following an examination of the conditions you want to improve and your anatomy. Read the questions on facelift and on liposuction for specific information on how these procedures relate to "lifting" a neck. In cases where liposuction alone can achieve your goals, a board-certified dermatologist with added training as a dermatologic surgeon and with experience in liposuction also may be an appropriate provider.

Improvement in the neck alone may make a remarkable difference in your appearance. You may find that you like wearing turtlenecks, because your neck no longer hangs over them. Conversely, if you have had plastymal bands in the neck corrected, you will no longer feel the need to hide behind turtlenecks or scarves. But the results of any procedure to correct the signs of aging in your neck are not permanent. You will continue to age naturally, however, from a now-much-younger starting point.

Note: Botox® therapy may be recommended with plastysmaplasty to relax the vertical banding muscles in the neck before surgical correction, or afterwards to better maintain the results of your neck lift.

75. Will it be obvious that I had plastic surgery to look younger?

Before the advent of SMAS lifts and limited incision brow lifts, surgical rejuvenation procedures were performed by tightly pulling back facial skin and then reducing excess skin. This sometimes produced a very obviously operated-on appearance. Even with SMAS and limited incision brow lifts, earlier trends in rejuvenation procedures over-corrected the conditions that contribute to an aging appearance. The assumption was that by over-correcting initially, the results of surgical rejuvenation would then last longer.

However, over-correction is no longer the trend or readily practiced by most plastic surgeons. Today, surgical advances in plastic surgery and refined techniques in rejuvenation procedures respond to the needs of individuals who want natural results, not an obviously operated-on appearance. This includes not only smoothing to achieve a lift, but also "filling"—replacing lost volume from the face through fat or other tissue grafting or by repositioning fat and muscle. The goal of surgical facial rejuvenation procedures is not a shrinking face that gets tighter and tighter with each procedure. Rather, it is to look like a more youthful version of yourself—soft, full, smooth, *and* with natural expressions and a natural appearance.

Further, rejuvenation procedures don't require over-correcting or "extra" tightening for results that last a decade. In fact, as you continue to age, the signs of aging may be visible sooner on a face that has had over-correction of the skin.

76. Are there alternatives to surgical rejuvenation of the face?

There are a number of alternatives to rejuvenative plastic surgery. The nonsurgical treatments do not, however, achieve the same end as do the surgical procedures discussed in this chapter. Nonsurgical rejuvenation and skin treatments may delay the need for surgical treatment, complement surgical rejuvenation, or prolong the outcomes of some surgical procedures. These treatments include Botox® therapy for wrinkle reduction and facial shaping, injectable fillers, and skin resurfacing. The following chapter focuses fully on these treatment categories and their role in plastic surgery, even though they are not considered surgical procedures.

77. Are there special considerations for men?

Men are currently a minority among patients undergoing surgical rejuvenation procedures, but they do total over 1.2 million aesthetic patients (including invasive and noninvasive procedures) as reported by the American Society of Plastic Surgeons in 2003. There are only a few special considerations for men, specifically related to the difference in male hair patterns.

The first consideration with facelift surgery is that facial hair may grow in the tragus (bulge in the front of the ear) or behind the ear following surgery. A man can elect to undergo laser hair removal following surgery or just be prepared to shave those regions as needed.

The second consideration is both with facelift and brow lift procedures and the visibility of scars in receding hairlines, thinning hair, or in a bald scalp. Limited incision techniques (such as an endoscopic brow lift versus coronal incision techniques) can reduce the amount of visible scars where appropriate. Scars should not, however, deter you from considering rejuvenative procedures, even if you are bald or balding. Rather, you should make your decision after consulting with a plastic surgeon experienced in facial rejuvenation who has additional experience in specifically treating the male patient.

Looking Younger: Surgical Facial Rejuvenation

PART ELEVEN

Plastic Surgery Without Surgery: Minimally Invasive Procedures

What are minimally invasive procedures?

What are Botox®, fillers, chemical peel, and dermabrasion procedures?

What are laser and radio wave treatments in plastic surgery?

How safe are minimally invasive procedures?

More ...

Nonsurgical and less invasive treatments used to improve appearance or delay the signs of aging are rising rapidly in consumer interest and demand. There are three categories of these minimally invasive treatments: injection therapies, soft tissue implants (also called fillers), and skin resurfacing. The procedures in these categories can soften or improve the signs of aging or heredity, but not with the same effect or outcomes as do surgically invasive procedures.

78. What are minimally invasive procedures?

Minimally invasive procedures are those treatments that address the skin and underlying tissue without major surgical intervention. The popularity of these procedures is growing rapidly in the United States. While minor in scope, these procedures can make a very visible improvement in your appearance. They offer high patient satisfaction, the lack of significant recovery time or discomfort, and a lower cost compared to traditional plastic surgery. However, there are two things you must understand:

- The results are not the same as those achieved with the surgical procedures.
- Although they are nonsurgical in most cases, these are, nonetheless, medical procedures that do carry the potential for risk.

Minimally invasive procedures fall under three specific categories:

- Injection therapies that change soft tissue function, namely Botox® Cosmetic therapy to soften existing wrinkles and facial folds;

- Soft issue augmentation (enhancement) with substances that are either injected or placed through limited surgical techniques (including pharmaceutical and your own tissues);
- Skin resurfacing techniques, including mechanical resurfacing, chemical resurfacing, and laser or light-based procedures.

Various combinations of these treatments are frequently used to complement or enhance the effects of one another. Multiple procedures can be staged (done in a series of treatments) or performed at the same time.

The most common combination of minimally invasive procedures is an injection of Botox® (to relax the muscles that produce an offending wrinkle) and an injection of a soft tissue filler (to further soften and smooth the appearance of the area). For example, if Botox® is injected to relax the vertical muscles that cause the grooves between your eyebrows, a soft tissue filler can be injected in those grooves at the same office visit to further enhance the result. Research indicates that when used together, the results of both of these treatments are enhanced and can last somewhat longer than if they were used independently.

You may also undergo mild resurfacing procedures, such as a light chemical peel or microdermabrasion, just prior to injection of Botox® or a filler. But you would not want to undergo any treatment that may apply pressure to or manipulate the skin following injection of Botox® or a filler. In addition, any minimally invasive treatment can be used to enhance the results of more invasive surgical procedures.

Plastic Surgery Without Surgery

There are numerous options in minimally invasive procedures. The treatments discussed in this chapter are commonly accepted practices in plastic surgery; the drugs and devices discussed are approved by the U.S. Food and Drug Administration (FDA). Some, however, only have off-label use, which means that the specific application for FDA approval of that drug or device has not yet been reviewed by the FDA. Further, the fact that a given treatment is FDA-approved does not mean you will always get the same results as those demonstrated in clinical studies.

Much of the success of these procedures is directly the result of the qualified providers administering treatment. Therefore, you should always first make certain that the surgeon or medical professional providing treatment is qualified and licensed.

79. Who should I choose to perform minimally invasive procedures?

In most states the only regulation is that minimally invasive procedures be performed in a licensed facility by a licensed medical professional. But not all states require that they be performed in a medical facility or that the medical professional administering treatment be a physician. You need to choose only a qualified, board-certified plastic surgeon, facial plastic surgeon, or dermatologist who is experienced specifically with the procedure in which you are interested. An ophthalmologist is also an appropriate provider for Botox® therapy around the eyes.

In some cases your treatment may be provided by a non-physician. Always be certain you have spoken with the practice's physician before your treatment and that the individual who will treat you is, in fact, a licensed medical professional under the supervision of a licensed, appropriately credentialed physician.

80. How can I stop my wrinkles or soften them?

Botox® is the brand name of a drug formulated from the natural proteins of botulinum toxin type A. Botox® Cosmetic is the form of this drug labeled and used for aesthetic reasons.

Botox® was initially developed and approved by the FDA in 1989 to treat severe muscle spasms or uncontrollable blinking in the eyes (blepharospasm) and misaligned eyes (strabismus). In 2000, Botox® was approved to treat a neurological disorder called cervical dystonia that causes severe neck and shoulder contractions. As a result of treatment of blepharospasm, the aesthetic benefits of Botox® were discovered. In 2002, Botox® Cosmetic was approved by the FDA specifically for the aesthetic benefits found when injected into the glabella region, which is the area where frown lines develop high on the bridge of the nose, between the eyebrows. Today, Botox® is safely used on an off-label basis to reduce crow's feet, horizontal brow furrows, and vertical banding of the neck. Some providers use Botox® to shape the appearance of the mid face and nasolabial region (from the nose to the outer corners of the mouth). There has been another brand of botulinum toxin marketed in the United States, but because of issues relating to the efficacy and outcomes, it is no longer marketed. As of the writing of this book (2004), Botox® is the only U.S.

Plastic Surgery Without Surgery

FDA-approved treatment of its kind. (A substance called Dysport® is pending FDA approval.)

Botox® specifically produces:

- A softening of the facial creases and folds that result when certain facial expressions are made
- A restored balance in cases of facial asymmetry due to unequal muscle action or inaction in the face

Botox® is appropriately administered only by specially trained, board-certified plastic surgeons, facial plastic surgeons, dermatologists, and in some cases ophthalmic plastic surgeons. However, when choosing a provider, not only is board-certification important, but equally important are that your provider:

- Has proof of formal training in Botox® Cosmetic therapy either from Allergan Inc. (the makers of Botox®) or from an accredited medical society as listed in Part 2 of this book
- Fully examines your facial anatomy and musculature before determining where and how much Botox® to inject
- Fully discloses all information to you about Botox® and secures your written consent
- Has taken a medical history, including a history of neurological disorders and allergies

Botox® injection is a very safe procedure in trained hands. Be careful when marketing messages of cheap treatment and deep discounts are given. Sometimes you may end up with highly diluted concentrations of Botox® that won't produce good outcomes, or it may leak to other areas and cause muscle weakness in the wrong place.

Are you covered?

Botox® is not reimbursed by insurers for use in facial rejuvenation.

Good candidates

Good candidates for Botox® therapy in facial rejuvenation are healthy adults with good muscle tone and skin elasticity who do not have neurologic disorders. Younger patients can benefit from Botox® therapy by preventing formation of deep creases and furrows in the upper third of the face. Those patients who already have these creases will see a marked improvement and smoother appearance of the region. Botox® does not treat visible wrinkles on the skin surface; it relaxes the underlying muscles that create these creases through repeated movement. Therefore, if the overlying skin has lost elasticity, a surgical lift may be a better option for you.

How it's done

Botox® treatment can be performed in a qualified provider's office examination room. A fine needle is used to inject Botox®, so icing may not be necessary but is offered for the comfort of some individuals. The area to be injected will be cleansed most commonly with alcohol. You will be asked to make certain expressions, and your surgeon may make marks on the skin at proposed injection sites. Depending on the area to be treated, you may receive a few or more injections in a given region to achieve your desired results. Botox® alone is not injected; it is diluted in very small amounts of saline. You will be told not to rub the area or to bend forward in the few hours following treatment so that the Botox® does not disperse to other muscles. You may later resume all normal activity. Know that you may have some bruising and will not see any obvious changes for several days following injection.

What to expect

Botox® works by blocking acetylcholine, a chemical released from nerve cells that facilitate muscle contraction. Within 5 to 14 days following treatment, Botox® will fully take effect and relax the muscles that were treated. By denervating those muscles, you will weaken the movements that cause the creases you are treating.

All of our anatomies differ, and some individuals may not get the desired outcome from the first treatment cycle with Botox®. Be certain to tell your provider if the initial treatment did not produce your desired results; the dosage of Botox® and your treatment may need to be modified.

It is advised to wait at least three months between treatment cycles of Botox®, because if you do it more often your body can produce antibodies that may make Botox® ineffective in the future. Botox® is not permanent, lasting from four to six months in most individuals. FDA guidelines state 120 days. If treatment is not repeated, the results of Botox® will diminish and your appearance will return to its original condition.

What you need to know

The risks of Botox® are few, and rare, when properly injected. Some individuals may experience a mild headache, others have mild flu-like symptoms in the few days following initial treatment; these are both uncommon. In addition, facial asymmetry, drooping eyelid, and even impaired vision are possible. These complications are temporary and highly unlikely in the hands of skilled providers. There is always the risk of infection at the injection sites, but this, too, is rare. Also, with injection in the neck, inability to swallow can be a rare and serious complication that may require surgical intervention.

Your responsibilities

Following all instructions immediately after treatment is imperative. In addition, you must follow up with your provider should your results not present as expected or if you experience any undesirable side effects.

Your results

For a very limited procedure that takes only a few moments to administer, Botox® can produce some visible improvements. It is also beneficial in refining and extending the results of many surgical procedures such as necklift and browlift. As you continue Botox® treatment, you may find a lengthening of the intervals between treatments. Because Botox® is completely eliminated from the body over time, if for some reason you do not like the results, they are not permanent and will gradually disappear.

81. Is Botox® really safe?

Consider that the average patient receives, in the forehead and glabella region, about 30 to 40 units of Botox® diluted in saline. Patients being medically treated for conditions such as cervical, laryngeal, and dystonias (uncontrolled spasms of shoulders and neck, larynx or voice box, and limbs), spasm following stroke, multiple sclerosis, and brain and spinal cord injury, receive doses that in many cases are in excess of 10 times the cosmetic dosages of Botox®. These dosages are not harmful or toxic to these patients—they are necessary to produce the desired outcome of treatment.

The toxicity limit of Botox® is defined as more than 1000 units in a single dose. Most physicians don't even have that much Botox® in their offices at one time.

When in the hands of a qualified provider, Botox® is absolutely safe. Even in off-label use, over 2.5 million people were treated with Botox® in the first year following FDA approval (as reported by Botox® manufacturer, Alleragan, Inc.). Of these cases there have been no U.S. FDA Medwatch publications indicating proper treatment compromised the health of a patient. The key here is proper treatment that requires, as noted above:

- An appropriately trained, board-certified plastic surgeon, facial plastic surgeon, dermatologist or ophthalmologist provider who is experienced in those areas that you wish to have treated.
- Initial complete analysis of your facial anatomy and muscle movements.
- Discussion of any medical conditions that may contraindicate the use of Botox®.
- Proper procedure of informed consent, including a discussion of possible sequelae.

82. Where can or should Botox® be used?

In 2002, the FDA approved Botox® for the glabella region, or frown lines between the brows. They did not review data on other facial regions. However, other regions commonly safely injected on an off-label basis (and appropriate to consider) include:

- The entire forehead, for horizontal furrows (although not immediately above the lateral brows)
- The region outside the eyes, to soften the angled creases that develop, called crow's feet

In addition, some plastic surgeons use Botox® to soften:

- Vertical muscle cords in the neck
- The nasolabial region, those lines from the nose to the outer corners of the mouth

These two treatment areas are not considered common practices. In addition, Botox® has been used to treat a condition called hyperhydrosis (excessive perspiration). It has also been used for "facial shaping," which improves asymmetry due to facial paralysis. Botox® can be injected in the upper or lower eyelid to reduce spasm, but not for cosmetic reasons. Ask your provider specifically about his or her experience in treating any one of these conditions.

Physical location

You need to pay attention to the setting in which the procedure is performed. Early in its introduction Botox® was injected into patients at "Botox® parties." Allergan, Inc., the manufacturer of Botox® Cosmetic, in a position statement released in 2002 regarding the promotion of Botox® Cosmetic, stated: "Botox® Cosmetic should be administered in a medically appropriate environment as deemed suitable by the authorized health care professional."

In addition, the medical societies of appropriate providers of Botox® therapy have been very vocal against treatment in settings such as "Botox® parties." Specifically, the American Society of Plastic Surgeons stated in April 2002: "The consumption of alcohol before, during, or after the medical procedure could affect a patient's decision and outcome. The decision to have a medical procedure should be made without the influence of alcohol or peer pressure."

The American Society for Dermatologic Surgery reported in their 2003 procedural nearly 500,000 patients treated with Botox® by their members in 2003.

All of the professional societies of qualified Botox® providers report steady increases in the rise of Botox® treatment since formal FDA approval, ranging from 30% to 50%. As well, Botox® is the leading nonsurgical aesthetic procedure among all of these groups.

In 2003, the American Society of Plastic Surgeons reported their surgeons to have treated nearly 2.9 million Botox® Cosmetic treatments. Botox® injections comprised 42% of all aesthetic plastic surgery procedures, of which 12% of patients were men.

In the same statement, the ASPS advised the public that those interested in Botox® should check the provider's credentials, seek a complete patient evaluation, be informed, and choose an appropriate setting.

83. How can I soften creases and wrinkles, or enhance the fullness of my face?

Soft tissue fillers are used to fill or soften irregular contours in the skin, or to create or restore volume underlying soft tissue. Fillers are technically implants or grafts used to enhance or modify the soft tissues, most commonly of the face. The variations include:

• Injectable pharmaceutical fillers
• Implanted pharmaceutical fillers
• Your own tissue (fat, dermis, or fascia), injected or implanted

In general, soft tissue fillers are used to:

• Fill fine lines, wrinkles, and deeper creases in the skin
• Restore or create fullness in the soft tissues under the skin
• Enhance the lips

- Improve the appearance of recessed or concave scars

They can be used alone, in combination with other minimally invasive procedures, or to further refine or enhance the outcomes of surgical procedures.

Pharmaceutical fillers are technically medical devices or implants, not drugs. Most soft tissue fillers are generally not permanent: the results of treatment will diminish over time. There are, however, some fillers that are considered semipermanent or permanent. What you need to consider is that our faces are always changing as the result of such things as aging and weight change. While the notion of a permanent filler may seem attractive, it may not be desirable or appropriate for the long term. You must carefully evaluate all of your options in soft tissue enhancement with a qualified provider. Your provider should take the time to fully review with you:

- Your facial anatomy and the improvement you desire
- Your options in appropriate fillers and possible alternatives to treat the conditions you wish to improve
- All the known immediate and long-term outcomes of the specific filler you are considering, including possible complications and risks
- Confirm your understanding and secure your consent through informed consent procedures

In addition, if you are going to have a pharmaceutical implant, be certain that the brand used is specifically named on any informed consent documents.

Much like Botox®, injectable pharmaceutical fillers are readily available, and there are many unqualified providers offering treatment. Often, these unqualified providers entice consumers with deep discounts, and in some cases treatment is provided with an unknown or imported substance that is not FDA approved. It is therefore important that you:

- Choose an appropriately trained, board-certified provider, namely a plastic surgeon, facial plastic surgeon, or dermatologist
- Accept treatment only of a brand-name injectable drug or filler substance that is approved in the United States by the FDA. Approval may be specific to your planned treatment or in readily accepted off-label use. Additionally, you may choose to be a patient in an approved, controlled research study for an injectable cosmetic drug under consideration for FDA approval.

Injectable and implanted fillers are most commonly used in the face, but they can also be used to soften the appearance of the back of the hands, and scars or skin irregularities anywhere on the body. However, they are not designed to be used in large areas, and outcomes, at present, are only reported for facial tissues. The results you get on your face might be very different from your hands, as skin on the back of the hands is thinner and looser than facial skin.

84. What are injectable pharmaceutical fillers?

Injectable pharmaceutical soft tissue fillers have been around for years, with the introduction of bovine-based (cow) collagen in the 1980s, now under the brand names Zyderm® and Zyplast®. The newer generation of facial fillers offers two significant advantages over bovine collagen:

- Some fillers are naturally derived and do not pose the risk of allergy as do those derived from animal sources
- Some offer results lasting 2 to 4 times longer than collagen

As of the writing of this book these fillers, by brand name, include:

Restylane®: Approved by the FDA in December 2003, it is a non-animal, stabilized hyaluronic acid (NASHA). Hyaluronic acid is a compound found in the skin of all humans and in many topical moisturizers. Other medical uses of hyaluronic acid-based pharmaceuticals include injection to increase the lubrication of joints where cartilage has diminished.

Restylane® is naturally derived and therefore it requires no pre-allergy testing. The results of Restylane® injections last from six months to as much as a year in some patients. Two additional formulations of Restylane® include:

- Restylane Fine Lines®, to fill fine lines in thinner tissues such as those surrounding the mouth and crows feet
- Perlane® a thicker formulation for deeper creases and areas of greater facial movement such as the nasolabial folds (the creases that run from the nose to the mouth)

Juvéderm™: The brand name of another non-animal stabilized formulation of hyaluronic acid. It was submitted for U.S. approval in late 2003 and as of the writing of this book has not yet received approval.

Hylaform®: Was approved by the FDA in April 2004. It is a cross-linked form of hyluronic acid derived from rooster combs. It can pose a risk of allergy, particularly in those individuals who have known allergies to birds or eggs. However no pre-allergy testing is required. Hylaform® comes in two formulations and is reported to last from four to six months, and in some cases even a bit longer.

Cosmoderm® and Cosmoplast®: Two formulations of collagen from human-derived sources that do not require pre-allergy testing and are suitable for all of the common conditions improved by injectable soft-tissue fillers. However, the duration of results for both of these fillers is typically two to three months, after which time all of the filler is absorbed by the body.

Radiance®: A filler that, as of the writing of this book, is used on an off-label basis. This means that it is approved by the U.S. FDA, but not specifically for aesthetic procedures. Radiance® is a form of hydroxyapetite, a substance found naturally in the bones of humans. It can be injected into the deeper soft tissues such as the nasolabial folds or the cheeks, to either fill deep creases or increase volume. It is reported to last from three to five years in some individuals. Because it is not a completely fluid substance, it does have the risk of clumping—the tiny granules in Radiance® can begin to clump together with repeated movement in areas where it is injected. In addition, Radiance® can migrate, or move from the area in which it was injected, generally gravitating downward in the soft tissues, creating an unnatural lump under the skin.

Sculptra®: Conditional approval was granted by the FDA in April 2004 to Sculptra®, a filler substance marketed as New-Fill in Europe, specifically to restore facial fullness to HIV patients with a condition called lipoatrophy (a wasting away of fat in the face that produces a drawn and very ill appearance). Sculptra® may be offered to healthy patients as a facial filler in off-label use. Like Radiance® and other more permanent fillers, Sculptra® carries the risk of clumping and the formation of granulomas in the skin. This is, in fact, because the substance is comprised of tiny crystals of polylactic acid (PLLA)—it is microscopically granular. When injected into the deeper layers of the soft tissue, collagen naturally begins to form around these crystals, thus increasing fullness in the soft tissue. A series of treatments at staged intervals of a few weeks to a month or more is required to achieve desired results over time, and the number of treatments required varies. Even though the filler is considered "semi-permanent," annual touch-ups may be necessary to maintain results once they are achieved.

Artecoll® or Artefill®: A formulation of collagen in which microscopic silicone beads are suspended. It was recommended for approval by an advisory panel to the U.S. FDA in February 2003; however, as of the writing of this book, it has not been formally approved. The principle of Artecoll® treatment is that as the collagen component of the filler is absorbed by the body, your own collagen will begin to form around the silicone beads that remain at the injected sites. This implies that Artecoll® may be a nearly permanent filler. However, complications as a result of clumping or migrating of those silicone beads have made Artecoll® a highly debated, and therefore very carefully reviewed, filler.

Are you covered?

Soft-tissue augmentation with injectable fillers is an aesthetic procedure and not eligible for insurance coverage.

Good candidates

Good candidates for soft-tissue fillers are healthy men and women of any age without active diseases of the skin and with good skin tone. These individuals accept that while soft-tissue fillers can remarkably improve fullness and create a smoother appearance in the skin, they are not a substitute for, and do not produce the same results as, surgical facial rejuvenation.

How it's done

Soft tissue filler injections are performed in your plastic surgeon's, facial plastic surgeon's, or dermatologist's office exam room. The area to be injected will be cleansed, most likely with alcohol. Depending on the filler and your comfort, a topical anesthetic cream may be applied and a local anesthetic agent injected to numb the region to be filled. Your physician may mark the regions to be filled.

Injections in multiple locations will be made to place the filler substance within the dermis of the skin, and in some cases even deeper into the soft tissues. Depending on the filler used, the area may be somewhat "over-filled" in the days immediately following treatment. The fluid or anesthetic added to some fillers will be absorbed and therefore influence your outcomes.

What to expect

Once the injections are completed, you may be given ice to minimize discomfort and possible swelling and bruising. You may be uncomfortable at the injection site but have no real physical impairment that would require restricted activity in any way following the procedure. Follow your physician's instructions regarding pressure or massage to the areas where filler has been placed.

Cosmetics will usually cover any swelling, redness, or bruising that appears for a few days following the procedure.

What you need to know

The risks and complications of injectable pharmaceutical fillers include those already described as well as local swelling, redness, and bruising at the injection sites. Infection is possible, but rare. If local anesthetic agents are used, there is also the possibility of a reaction to these anesthetics. In addition, some filler substances may not be appropriate on darkly pigmented or African-American patients. If you are an individual of color, make certain your provider states specifically that the filler recommended in your case is appropriate.

Your obligations

Clearly defining all known allergies and following all of your provider's instructions are important to achieve a safe and good result from treatment with injectable fillers.

Your goals, now and in the future

Injectable soft-tissue fillers can provide dramatic changes in appearance, or simply enhance and soften facial features. Results vary in duration based on the filler used. Once the filler is fully absorbed, your appearance will return to its previous condition, if you choose not to repeat treatment to maintain your outcomes. Only where facial structures are excessively over-filled for long periods of time, and where skin has poor elasticity, can there be a slight increase in sagging once the filler has been fully absorbed.

In 2003, soft-tissue augmentation, specifically collagen injection and Restylane®, was reported by the American Society of Plastic Surgeons to number just over 521,000 procedures, whereas in 2001 nearly 800,000 procedures were performed. The American Society for Dermatologic Surgeons reported over 206,000 procedures in 2002. Radiance® injections numbered nearly 62,000 in 2003.

It can be predicted that in 2004, the number of procedures performed with injectable soft-tissue fillers will skyrocket, nearly as much or more than it did after Botox® approval by the FDA in 2002. Why? Although fillers have existed for some time, the new generation of fillers is superior to bovine collagen: they last longer and have fewer allergy concerns. People want to look better without a prolonged recovery, surgical pain, or deep hole in their pocket.

85. What are minimally invasive implanted fillers?

Implanted pharmaceutical fillers are sheet, cylindrical, or fabric-like medical devices that enhance soft tissues. The implants are placed through small incisions during "minimally invasive" surgery. Procedures are most commonly performed using local anesthetic agents, sometimes in conjunction with oral sedation. The commonly implanted fillers include:

Absorbable implants: Alloderm and Dermaplant are sheet forms of collagen, a homogenized matrix of human tissue taken from cadavers. When used to augment soft tissues, namely the lips, an implant is surgically placed through incisions. It is as soft and pliable as one's own tissue. Because these implants are derived from human sources, there is no risk of allergy.

Alloderm® and Dermaplant® absorb more slowly than some injectable fillers. But they do lose volume over time. Some patients' results last as little as six months, while others may last a year or more.

In addition, there is an injectable form of Alloderm®, called Cymetra®, which is injected in the deep layer of the dermis (skin), or just below that layer. Note that implantable fillers placed under the skin results in a change to the structure of underlying soft tissues, whereas injectable fillers change the nature of skin itself.

Permanent Implants (strands): Polytetrafluoroethylene (ePTFE) is a synthetic polyester material that was introduced in the 1990s by plastic surgeons to permanently augment soft tissues. The strands are pliable, although not the same texture as human tissue. Therefore, some patients find them awkward and stiff when implanted.

ePTFE is permanent and cannot be absorbed by your body. However, as you age and naturally lose facial volume, the strands may become apparent on the surface of your skin. Much like any foreign implanted structure in the body, there is the risk of developing irregularly firm tissue over the implant that may require removal or replacement.

There are different brands of ePTFE. Gortex® (by Gore) was the first, most commonly used, brand. There are newer brands (such as Advanta®) that are softer and more porous. They may feel more natural but are more difficult to remove if there is a complication. All of these strands are cylindrical and can be placed through small stab incisions. They are different from the larger, structural implants (like cheek and chin implants) that require true surgical placement.

What you need to know

The cost and the recovery time of implanted pharmaceutical fillers are greater than procedures using injected pharmaceutical fillers. For example, the cost of a lip augmentation with an implanted material may be three to four times greater than if the procedures were performed using an injectable filler. The process of placing the implant can result in greater swelling, bruising, and discomfort than injections, requiring as much as a week for recovery. However, permanent implantable fillers may preclude the need for multiple, continued injections. Again, know your alternatives and how you want to proceed. Many people opt for shorter-term injections first, to see if they like the results. Then they gradually work their way up to more invasive, more long-lasting treatments.

In 2003, the American Society of Plastic Surgeons reported lip augmentation with materials other than injectable materials at nearly 23,000 procedures.

86. How are my own fat and other tissues used as fillers?

Your own tissues may be used as injectable or implantable fillers. The most common form is fat. It is frequently used when removed during a given procedure and then placed in another location where a filler is needed. This technique is called "fat grafting" and is very helpful in facial rejuvenation procedures.

For example, during eyelid surgery, the fat under your lower eyelid may be bulging into skin, causing excess bagginess while the area underneath is hollow (tear trough deformity). To remove that fat would result in an even worse condition—a thin loose bag that is sunken-in. By redistributing that fat either by a graft or flap (leaving it attached to its blood supply but changing its location) a smooth, youthful contour may be created.

In a different application, your own tissue can be removed from an area of the body (during liposuction, for example) and then used to soften areas in the face or other parts of the body. In this case, the fat is injected, not grafted.

Autologous fat injections, fat transfer, or micro-lipoinjection are terms used to define injectable soft tissue augmentation that uses one's own fat instead of pharmaceutical fillers. Typically, the fat is extracted from the abdomen, buttocks, or thighs through lipo-suction techniques. A cannula or a large needle attached to a syringe will extract the fat. Once removed, the fat is processed and then reinjected. Fat may also be frozen and stored for future use.

What you need to know

The differences between injections of your own fat and those of pharmaceutical fillers include:

- There is no chance of allergic reaction to your own fat because it is taken from your body.
- There is a reported higher level of discomfort with fat injections, as human fat has less fluid than phar-maceutical substances. There is also a longer period of swelling and bruising following treatment.
- Because of the higher level of discomfort, anesthetic agents must be used.
- Because of irregular absorption and added anes-thetic agents required, the areas to be corrected

must be "over-filled." The amount of fat reabsorbed over the following months cannot be predetermined. Therefore, outcomes with human fat seem to be less predictable than with many of the injectable pharmaceutical fillers.

• Multiple treatments may be required to achieve long-lasting results.

Implanted soft tissue (grafts)

Human tissue, such as fat, dermis, or fascia, can also be grafted to augment soft tissues. Fat or dermis can be removed from distant or local areas and then implanted in areas of the face as needed. Fascia is a layer of tissue, primarily composed of collagen, that covers the muscles. This is very vascular and very hearty thin tissue that can be used to soften many creases or thinned areas of the skin to improve contour. Fat, dermis, and fascia can be used to fill deeper defects or enhance fullness in the facial features as well. Soft tissue may be grafted as an isolated procedure, or more commonly, it may be used in conjunction with facial rejuvenation surgery when the donor tissue is readily available.

> The American Society of Plastic Surgeons reports nearly 62,000 fat injection procedures in 2003, the American Society for Aesthetic Plastic Surgery nearly 90,000 procedures in the same year, and the American Society for Dermatologic Surgery about 22,000 procedures of autologous fat injection in 2003.

87. What is skin resurfacing?

Skin resurfacing is the third category of noninvasive procedures. Skin resurfacing procedures remove the epidermis and superficial dermis (upper layers) of the skin. They may also change the nature of the remaining skin by altering the components of the dermis. Human skin naturally renews itself on a regular basis, shedding the top layer of dead, often keratinized cells and allows new cells to rise to the skin surface. While skin resurfacing procedures are more commonly performed on facial skin, they can be performed anywhere on the body. However, not all procedures are appropriate for treatment of the delicate skin of the neck.

Resurfacing procedures speed the process of skin renewal, and some procedures will change the texture of the skin as well. There are different degrees of resurfacing treatment:

1. Light resurfacing can refresh the skin's appearance and improve skin health by exfoliating the skin. It removes the dead, and often rough, top layer of cells that can clog pores and inhibit oxygen from reaching healthy cells. It can also clear congested and enlarged pores that are more likely to develop acne pimples, pustules, and cysts. Light exfoliation treatments include milder chemical peels and mechanical exfoliations through microdermabrasion.

2. Deeper resurfacing can stimulate faster cell renewal, particularly in aging skin that does not naturally renew as quickly. It can also ablate (remove the outer layers of the skin) and change underlying collagen. Procedures include deeper chemical peels, mechanical resurfacing such as dermabrasion or dermaplaning, and some laser procedures (such as Erbium Yag, and CO_2).

3. Dermal change techniques include light and soundwave based procedures. These techniques are thought to change the collagen and change the texture of the skin. The outer layer (epidermis) is not affected, so

The American Society for Dermatologic Surgery reports over 420,000 resurfacing procedures performed by their members in 2003. The American Society of Plastic Surgeons reports on these procedures individually.

recovery is minimal. But the results are not as dramatic as with the deeper resurfacing techniques.

88. What are chemical peels?

Chemical peels are treatments that apply topical chemicals to the skin to resurface the skin in varying degrees. The least invasive peels include glycolic, or alpha hydroxy acid peels, in varying concentrations. Beta hydroxy, tretinoin (or vitamin A based) peels and Jessner's peels are somewhat deeper. The most invasive peels that should only be performed by a board-certified plastic surgeon, facial plastic surgeon or dermatologist include phenol and trichloroacetic acid or TCA peels.

Noninvasive peels will exfoliate skin to refresh and soften it without creating any wounds. With repeated treatments these may improve skin tone and fine lines. In general, noninvasive peels are administered by a licensed esthetician (one who provides nonmedical care of the skin in the health and beauty industry) or specially trained nurse in a board-certified physician's office. (The skin peels offered in a non-physician-based setting are usually state-regulated at a much lower concentration.) These types of peels are purely aesthetic and are not reimbursable by insurance.

Good candidates

Noninvasive peels can benefit nearly every type of skin. However, both the type of peel that is right for you and the frequency of treatments are highly variable. Treatment should be based on your preference, your skin condition and color, and your goals. Anyone considering a peel of any kind should first consult with an appropriately credentialed and trained provider to evaluate your skin, and then discuss treatment options.

How it's done

Noninvasive or mild peels are performed in a physician's office exam room or adjacent clinical skin care setting. The skin is first cleansed, then the peeling solution applied. The most common noninvasive peels include:

- Alpha-hydroxy glycolic formulations that range from 30% to as high as 70%
- Beta hydroxy peels, which are typically measured as levels 1 through 3 (3 being the more intense peel)
- Trentinoin peels, which vary from 3% to 8%

Some peels are self-neutralizing. The others are neutralized (or cleansed) from the skin a few moments following application. In many cases, the results of noninvasive peels are immediate—a fresher, clearer complexion that is bright and toned. In other cases, your skin may mildly peel over the following days to reveal your refreshed complexion.

What you need to know

There are noninvasive peels appropriate for nearly every skin type and color. The key to a good outcome is first careful analysis by a trained professional and, much like any plastic surgery procedure, complete education and informed consent. For example, no pregnant or nursing mother should undergo a peel using a treninoin- or vitamin A-based solution. In addition, while these peels are very safe in trained hands, there is always the possibility that skin can react adversely. Therefore, it is always advised that you choose a facility where a physician is on site during any treatment times.

Plastic Surgery Without Surgery

Your obligations

Diligent sun protection for several days following your peel is advised, as your refreshed skin is more susceptible to sun damage.

Your goals

Noninvasive peels will not produce immediate, dramatic changes in the skin. Rather, they will immediately produce softer, refreshed skin. Over time, with repeated procedures, you will notice more visible changes in softening of fine lines, correction of irregular pigmentation, and better skin tone.

Ironically, invasive peels were first developed and used by plastic surgeons and dermatologists to improve the appearance of wrinkles, acne, and other scarring on the surface of the skin. Phenol peels have been used since the 1980s; however, they are rarely used today. While phenol produces a very deeply penetrating peel, it can completely de-pigment skin (remove its color) and leave a very visible demarcation where it has been applied.

Trichloroacetic acid (TCA) peels were introduced at about the same time as phenol peels. The TCA peel is still used by plastic surgeons and dermatologists. It can effectively reduce surface wrinkling of the skin, and soften acne and other scars. In some cases, TCA peels are used to treat pigment disorders of the skin including freckles, age spots, and sun damage. In addition, TCA peels can be used to treat precancerous skin lesions, and these cases may be eligible for insurance reimbursement; precertification is always required.

Good candidates

Candidates for TCA peels must be healthy individuals without acute heart conditions or diseases that may impair healing. In addition, individuals with some forms of active skin disease in the areas to be treated must have those conditions controlled prior to treatment. Individuals with darker complexions may not be good candidates for invasive peels.

How it's done

A TCA peel should only be administered by a board-certified plastic surgeon, facial plastic surgeon, or dermatologist who is specifically trained in chemical resurfacing treatments of the skin. Treatment is performed in your physician's office. Your skin will first be cleansed, then the peeling solution in concentrations from 10% to 35% or more is applied. You will be carefully monitored as the peeling solution penetrates to the desired depth. Your skin will turn white or "frost" as the peel penetrates and lifts the skin surface. Once the peel is neutralized, ointment will be applied, and perhaps even dressings, to cover the very raw, red skin. Depending on the intensity of your peel, you may be swollen and feel very itchy for several days following the peel. You might find that sleeping with your head elevated will reduce the swelling you experience.

What to expect

Your skin will take from 5 to 10 days to heal initially. Very intense peels may require even longer healing periods. During the healing process, you will probably be given special ointment to keep your skin moist and will be advised to avoid pressing the telephone against your face, sleeping on your face, or touching your face unless necessary. Within two to three weeks all the crusting or scabs on your skin should resolve.

Within six to eight weeks your skin should return to a more normal hue, with a much-improved, smoother, better-toned appearance. It is imperative to protect your skin from the sun.

What you need to know

Some patients may develop scarring; others have irregular pigment or lack of pigment in the skin following an invasive peel.

Your obligations

Following all instructions to cleanse and care for your skin in the days and weeks following your peel is essential to a good outcome. You must continue sun protection for at least a year following your peel. Good sun protection is always sensible to practice.

The American Society of Plastic Surgeons reports over 995,000 chemical peels performed in ASPS-member plastic surgeons' offices in 2003.

What you will see

The results of invasive peels can dramatically improve the appearance of superficial fine lines and skin irregularities, including pigment and scarring. However, deeper wrinkles, scars, and pervasive pigmentation conditions, such as melasma, may only improve slightly. Skin will continue to age, and if you do not regularly practice good sun protection, your skin will readily show signs of sun damage.

89. What is dermabrasion?

Dermabrasion is a mechanical resurfacing of the skin that, much like chemical peels, can be noninvasive or mild, or can be invasive and fully ablate (remove) the skin's outer surface. The most common non-invasive form is microdermabrasion. More invasive forms of mechanical resurfacing are dermaplaning and dermabrasion

Microdermabrasion

Microdermabrasion is generally a noninvasive mechanical means of skin resurfacing. Fine crystals or particles are infused over the skin and immediately suctioned to lift the top layer of skin cells and decongest clogged pores. The amount of crystal flow and level of suction are variable and can range from very mild for more sensitive skin types to very aggressive for skin types that are able to tolerate the treatment. Microdermabrasion is used to deeply exfoliate the top layers of the skin dermis. The result is:

- Clearer, brighter skin
- More even skin tone
- Softening of irregular pigment following multiple treatments
- Softening of fine lines following multiple treatments

Microdermabrasion can accelerate skin cell renewal that, over time and repeated treatments, produces firmer, rejuvenated skin.

Microdermabrasion is best performed by a specially trained, licensed aesthetician or nurse in a medical setting, supervised by a board-certified plastic surgeon,

Plastic Surgery Without Surgery

facial plastic surgeon, or dermatologist. Microdermabrasion equipment is sold to non-physicians in most states, but is regulated at a much lower strength compared to the equipment available in a physician's office-based skin care facility or a physician's office.

Are you covered?

When prescribed by a dermatologist to treat active acne, microdermabrasion may be eligible for insurance coverage. Precertification is required.

Good candidates

Healthy individuals from adolescents through adulthood, without excessive skin sensitivities, are good candidates for microdermabrasion. Individuals with darker complexions should be cautious of the potential for existing pigmentation problems to worsen in some cases.

How it's done

Prior to microdermabrasion your skin will be cleansed and will be prepped with alcohol or a special toner to be certain it is free of any oils. Working on one region of the face at a time, the provider will place a glass wand on the face and move it back and forth in a controlled motion and pattern. The wand is attached to tubing through which crystals flow onto the face. These crystals loosen and exfoliate the surface skin cells. Simultaneous suction removes the crystals and removes dead skin cells and other matter clogging the pores.

Once treatment is completed, any excess crystals will be cleansed from the skin and appropriate hydration will be applied.

What to expect

You may have a slight redness for a few hours or days following microdermabrasion. It is imperative that you use sun protection at all times, as your skin is more susceptible to sun damage and sunburn. Improvement in overall skin clarity and pore congestion is visible almost immediately. Over the next few days your skin will be fully refreshed, clearer, and more vibrant.

Risks and complications

When performed by appropriately trained providers in an appropriate physician-based setting, microdermabrasion is a very safe procedure. Microdermabrasion can result in skin irritation, and in some cases, minor abrasions to the skin surface that should resolve within a few days of treatment. If the microdermabrasion wand is left stationary on any portion of skin, it may produce a small red lesion or bruise. Some individuals with asthma are sensitive to the crystal flow and may have some difficulty breathing during or immediately following treatment. If proper sanitation is not practiced (such as crystal recycling or wands not properly sanitized) there is the potential to develop skin infection.

Your obligations

Diligent sun protection for several days following your peel is advised, as your refreshed skin is more susceptible to sun damage. Also, be candid with your provider about all of your medical conditions and any discomfort you experience during treatment. Following the instructions, or schedule for treatment, recommended by your plastic surgeon or dermatologist is essential to achieving your goals.

What you will see and feel

The American Society of Plastic Surgeons reports nearly 936,000 microdermabrasion procedures performed in their member's offices in 2003.

Microdermabrasion produces immediate exfoliation and decongestion of the skin. Additional benefits are most effective when the procedure is performed in cycles, with several procedures being performed at specific intervals. Once your desired improvement is achieved, regular treatments can maintain your results and refresh your skin. Microdermabrasion has been shown to stimulate collagen growth in the dermis and increase natural collagen production. This can result in an improved skin tone, as well as clarity.

Dermabrasion and dermaplaning

Dermabrasion and dermaplaning are the first generation of mechanical skin resurfacing procedures. These treatments are very effective in improving the surface appearance of acne-scarred skin, fine wrinkles, and/or other visible irregularities of the skin.

Dermabrasion uses a mechanically held burr, typically of diamond particles, that rotates on the surface of the skin, literally polishing it away. The procedure requires local anesthesia, and in many cases, sedation. It produces wounds of varying depth that require special postoperative care to scab over and appropriately heal.

Dermaplaning resurfaces the skin with a rotating surgical blade called a dermatome, or by a hand-held surgical scalpel. The blade scrapes away the upper levels of the dermis. Dermaplaning also requires local anesthesia. In most cases sedation is also offered for your comfort.

During the course of healing from either dermabrasion or dermaplaning your activities will be restricted. You

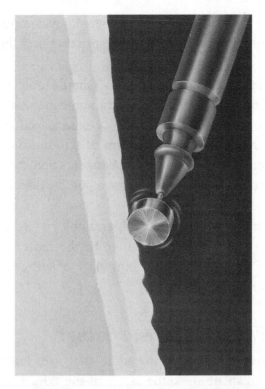

Figure 14   Dermabrasion. This is an artist's rendering and does not represent actual patient results. Individual results may vary. Courtesy of the American Society of Plastic Surgeons®. All rights reserved. Learn more at *www.plasticsurgery.org.*

must be fully protected from sunlight and take proper care of your skin. The success of your outcomes requires that you carefully follow all of the instructions for wound care. Either procedure can result in scarring and irregular pigmentation. Very careful examination of appropriate skin types, skin condition, and overall health are important to a successful outcome. In addition, because of the large wounds created by dermabrasion and dermaplaning, infection is possible, and you must be carefully monitored to avoid any complication that could result in a disfiguring appearance of the skin.

Dermabrasion, or dermaplaning, should only be performed by a board-certified plastic surgeon, facial plastic surgeon, or dermatologist who is experienced in these procedures as well as other forms of skin resurfacing. In your consultation, alternative treatments and the potential outcomes and complications should be discussed.

The American Society for Dermatologic Surgery in 2003 reported chemical peels to be the most common form of skin resurfacing, being 41% of all resurfacing procedures performed.

90. What is laser resurfacing?

Laser resurfacing is a procedure that uses laser technology to ablate the outer layers of the skin. Time may also change the collagen in the remaining adjacent dermis. Ablative lasers are direct beams of light that move over the skin's surface to destroy some cells. This allows for regeneration of new cells and creates a fresher, smoother appearance.

Use of an ablative laser, in controlled depths, can improve many surface conditions of the skin:

- Erase fine lines on the skin surface
- Soften deeper wrinkles and facial creases
- Reduce irregular pigment and brown spots
- Improve an uneven, blotchy appearance of the skin
- Improve the condition of uneven, scarred skin
- Tighten thinner skin that has lost elasticity, including skin of the lower eyelid

The American Society for Aesthetic Plastic Surgery reported nearly 28,000 dermabrasion procedures and over 858,000 microdermabrasion procedures in 2003.

Are you covered

Insurance coverage is sometimes provided for skin resurfacing with lasers when performed to treat precancerous skin lesions. Precertification is always necessary.

Good candidates

Good candidates for laser resurfacing are healthy individuals with realistic goals and with the time to invest in proper recovery from laser resurfacing. In addition, individuals with active skin diseases, such as acne, should have those conditions treated before undergoing laser resurfacing. Some types of lasers may not be appropriate for darker complexions.

How it's done

Laser resurfacing is an outpatient procedure that may be performed in an outpatient medical facility or in a physician's exam room when only small areas of the face are treated. Depending on the extent of your resurfacing procedure, you may have a local anesthetic with or without sedation. In cases where laser resurfacing is performed in conjunction with some surgical procedures, you may require general anesthesia. The

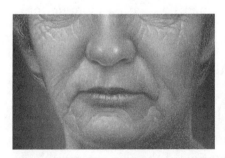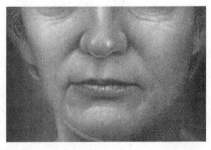

Figure 15   Laser resurfacing before and after. This is an artist's rendering and does not represent actual patient results. Individual results may vary. Courtesy of the American Society of Plastic Surgeons®. All rights reserved. Learn more at *www.plasticsurgery.org*.

areas to be treated will be cleansed with an antiseptic, and your eyes will be protected.

Using controlled movements of the laser on the skin surface, your physician will ablate, or destroy, layers of the skin to reach the desired depth of the dermis. Once the procedure is completed, your skin will be covered with special ointment and may be further covered with dressings.

What to expect

Following laser resurfacing you may be somewhat swollen in the treated region. Your skin will be red, raw, and may be sensitive or itch. As healing progresses, you may form crusts or scabs. You should be very gentle when cleansing and follow all instructions for postoperative care as directed by your physician. Dislodging or removing a crust too soon may result in scarring or hyperpigmentation. As you heal, you may find the newly formed skin is quite pink and sensitive. It is imperative that you protect your skin at all times from sun exposure, wind, and any form of irritation.

Within two to three weeks your results will be apparent: smoother, better-toned skin with a more uniform texture and color. However, it may take several more weeks or months for your skin to fully return to your more natural color and for all redness to subside.

What you need to know

Severe burns, infection, scarring, and hyper (darker) or hypo (lighter) pigmentation of the skin are possible. If you develop a rash or acne, notify your physician—topical treatments may need to be changed. The risks of skin resurfacing are minimized when a qualified and experienced board-certified plastic surgeon, facial plastic surgeon, or dermatologist performs your procedure and with proper post-resurfacing care.

Your obligations

Following all postoperative instructions, including proper wound care and sun protection, is essential to a good outcome. Ongoing skin care and sun protection are essential to maintaining that outcome as your skin naturally continues to age.

What you will see and feel

When performed to improve scarring, laser resurfacing is permanent as long as the condition that produced the scarring, such as acne, is under control. However, you may need several treatments, and the scar will not be completely removed. The results will include fewer shadows and less irregularity of the skin surface.

When performed to correct pigmentation disorders, laser resurfacing may produce permanent results. Brown spots can, however, recur. Sun exposure must be avoided to maintain your results. When used to refine wrinkling or improve loose sagging skin, results are also permanent, but your skin will continue to age naturally.

91. Are there other uses for lasers in plastic surgery?

In addition to ablative lasers for skin resurfacing, there are non-ablative lasers used in plastic surgery to change the nature of skin. These lasers have a single light source designed to penetrate the skin surface without removing or injuring it. The light source

The American Society of Plastic Surgeons reports nearly 181,000 laser resurfacing procedures in 2003.

changes the nature of skin. Each source or form of light is targeted to treat specific conditions.

Non-ablative lasers are most commonly used for:

- Rejuvenation of the skin for improved tone and elasticity
- Correction of pigmentation problems
- Correction of vascular problems such as veins, irregular blood vessels, and vascular lesions such as hemangiomas (tiny blood-filled beauty marks) or birthmarks
- Treatment of skin disorders such as acne
- Permanent hair removal
- Tattoo removal

It is unfortunate that tattoos have become fashionable, because frequently styles change. Even the most sophisticated means to remove tattoos result in either scars or irregular pigmentation of the skin. But not all tattoos are fashion statements, nor are they voluntary. A traumatic tattoo is one where skin discoloration occurs as particles of debris are forced under the skin during trauma, such as a severe abrasion on dirty concrete. These, too, can be very difficult to remove. In some cultures tattooing is a rite of passage to adulthood, and some children receive tattoos without their consent. In our own urban culture, tattoos can be gang symbols whose visibility may put a former gang member at risk, for life.

The American Society for Dermatologic Surgery reports that in 2003, 9% of more than 900,000 laser and light-based procedures performed by their members were tattoo removal.

Sclerotherapy can also be used for visible veins (spider veins) on the legs. It is an injection therapy that seals off offending veins. The veins then are no longer visible on the skin's surface. Brown spots and ulceration of the skin may occur. In general, your results will appear within a week to 10 days following treatment. It is important to know that leg veins can be an indication of underlying health conditions and, therefore, you should first consult with a vascular specialist before treating vessels larger than spider veins of the legs.

Are you covered?

Insurance coverage for treatment of some birthmarks and acne may be available. You should always check with your insurer.

Good candidates

Good candidates for non-ablative light-based treatments are healthy individuals with realistic goals and the patience to undergo multiple treatment cycles to achieve those goals. Individuals with skin sensitivities should disclose and discuss their conditions before undergoing any form of laser or light-based treatment. In addition, some forms of non-ablative light-based treatment may not be appropriate for darker complexions.

How it's done

Individual laser procedures vary in actual treatment. In general, your skin will be cleansed, and a cooling gel or topical anesthetic may be applied for your comfort. Your eyes will be protected. Only the areas to be treated are in contact with the light source emitted from the laser. In general, non-ablative lasers produce the following:

- When treating pigmentation, the treated areas may darken or scab immediately following your procedure. Over the next few days, crusts may shed, leaving pink new skin. You may then need to treat the skin with lightening gels to prevent the pigment from reoccurring.
- Treatment of vascular conditions, such as spider veins and hemangiomas, constricts the vessels that contribute to these problems. Initially you may have dark red or purple streaks. The areas will then gradually lighten. Multiple treatments may be necessary.
- When used for rejuvenation, a non-ablative laser stimulates collagen production deep beneath the skin. Over the few months following treatment, skin may feel and appear more firm. Multiple treatments may be necessary.
- Acne treatment with non-ablative lasers destroys the acne-causing bacteria deep beneath the skin. Over the days following treatment, existing pimples and pustules will diminish or shrink, and the ability of new pimples to form is greatly reduced.
- Hair removal is achieved when the light source form the laser reaches the hair follicle and seals it. However, because hair grows in cycles, it may take multiple cycles to achieve results.
- Tattoo removal requires multiple cycles to break up the pigment beneath the skin so that it may be naturally absorbed or exfoliated. All procedures to remove any type of tattoo will leave either some form of scarring or irregular pigment. Ironically, it is the more fair skin types with the darkest pigment in a tattoo that will likely have the better outcome after removal. Fair skin is less likely to show hypopigmentation (whitening) from laser treatment.

What you need to know

Because light emits heat, some individuals may experience mild surface burns from non-ablative laser treatments. In addition, the results are not fully predictable. Many individuals react differently to treatment. In the case of treating pigmentation disorders, there is the potential for pigment to worsen rather than improve. There is also the risk of hypopigmentation (whitening). A complete evaluation of your overall condition by a qualified provider is essential to achieving your goals. Also, non-ablative rejuvenative lasers generally do not produce immediate results. In fact, the only thing you may experience immediately following treatment is a slight tingling or redness, much like that of a sunburn.

92. Is there anything I need to know about the safety of lasers?

Medical devices such as lasers and light-based devices are regulated by the U.S. Food and Drug Administration. But the medical providers who use lasers and light-based devices are not regulated. Any licensed physician can purchase or lease a laser and perform resurfacing or other procedures. The success of your procedure and your safety are dependent on your choosing a qualified provider who is experienced with laser and light-based treatments. Only a board-certified plastic surgeon, facial plastic surgeon, or dermatologist should perform ablative laser procedures (those that remove layers of skin). Specially trained licensed medical professionals, in the offices of these providers, may perform non-ablative laser or light-based procedures. However, for your safety, there should always be a board-certified physician on site in the facility where you are being treated.

The American Society for Dermatologic Surgery reports nearly 730,000 laser and light-based procedures performed by their members or in their member's offices in 2003.

Non-ablative light-based treatments should not injure the skin surface; however, burns are an associated risk. Therefore, these non-ablative treatments are best provided by a board-certified plastic surgeon, facial plastic surgeon, or dermatologist. Specially trained nurses and physician's assistants are appropriate providers of photo-light and IPL treatments, but for your safety, one of the above-named physicians should be on premises in the office location where you are being treated.

93. What are radio wave treatments?

Over time, there have been many new devices tested and even approved by the U.S. FDA to rejuvenate the skin. Various non-ablative lasers and radio wave treatments are among the current devices being tested and marketed. In 2002, the U.S. FDA approved Thermacool™, a radio wave device to treat the wrinkles around the eyes by lifting and tightening sagging skin. Thermacool™ also has been used off-label on other regions of the face including the brow and nasolabial region. Radiofrequency does not react to pigment the way laser treatments do. Therefore, candidates for these treatments are not restricted to those with fair complexions.

Just how much improvement patients see from radio wave treatment, much like some non-ablative lasers, is variable. Any amount of "lift" is measured in millimeters and is generally seen only after multiple procedures and many months. In addition, radio wave treatment can be very uncomfortable.

If you are considering radiofrequency rejuvenation, be advised that no one with a pacemaker should undergo this treatment. Furthermore, results are not as apparent as with resurfacing procedures, and treatments may add up in cost. Know your options before making your decision.

Like any medical device, Thermacool™ is approved by the U.S. FDA, but users are not regulated. Therefore, if you are considering or wish to learn more about radiofrequency procedures, consult only with a board-certified plastic surgeon, facial plastic surgeon, or derma-tologist who has had specific training in this treatment.

Plastic Surgery Without Surgery

PART TWELVE

Recovery and Outcomes

What are the potential complications
of plastic surgery?

Can pain be controlled?

Can the signs of plastic surgery be camouflaged?

Can procedures be repeated?

More ...

Every medical treatment includes three very specific variables: recovery, risk, and outcomes.

Overall risk has been discussed in Part 5. In addition, after the description of each procedure, the possible complications and risks have been defined in each procedural question in this book. While recovery and outcomes have been discussed with each procedure, there is more you need to know.

Recovery includes both physical and emotional changes. Physical recovery can be as simple as an injection taking effect. Alternatively, recovery can require a recuperation period that may last months. During the various stages of physical recovery, your feelings about your decision to undergo plastic surgery will also change.

Outcomes are more than just the physical results of surgery. Outcomes include your level of satisfaction. Outcomes may also include the effect plastic surgery has on your relationships with others and on your life in general.

94. Why are complications, recovery, and outcomes always stated in variables?

Each individual responds differently to a given treatment. No procedure is performed identically on all patients.

The risks and complications in this book are defined in general terms. You may develop few—or possibly none—of these. However, you also could experience serious complications that are not listed in this book. Your chance of developing any complications is primarily dependent upon your health, your provider, and how you carry out your patient obligations. Know that medicine is not an exact science; unpredictable circumstances can present themselves in any form of medical treatment, not just plastic surgery.

For the same reason, we cannot be precise about the stages of recovery and about final outcomes. A given procedure is not performed exactly the same way, or to the same extent, on different individuals, because their anatomy and degree of deformity are different. Similarly, different people do not heal at the same rate, because their rebuilding systems are different. But your emotional preparedness does play an important part in your recovery and in your adaptation to your physical outcome.

You may question your decision to undergo plastic surgery in those first few days of recovery following an extensive procedure. A few weeks later, as recovery progresses, your thinking will begin to change. And, when you achieve your goals, you probably will have forgotten the negative aspects of the experience and will be enjoying the new you.

95. Can pain be controlled?

You need to accept the reality that some discomfort will be experienced. Pain management is an important part of plastic surgery. Your plastic surgeon should be candid with you about the pain that you are likely to experience and discuss the various means to control that pain. And you need to directly share your ability to cope with pain and your pain thresholds with your plastic surgeon. There are a variety of over-the-counter and prescription methods of reducing pain, but some may cause nausea after surgery and may need to be readjusted. Additionally, it is important to surround yourself with things and people that comfort you. Place yourself in an environment of serenity, and put aside anything (or anyone) that causes you stress.

In the procedural descriptions, we have stated that a responsible adult friend, family member, or caregiver should be with you following the procedure. This person should not only care for your safety, but also support your decision to have surgery and be prepared to nurture you in a way that makes you feel comfortable. You may or may not want to have someone fussing over you—straightening pillows, changing dressings, or making you milkshakes. But you must have someone assist and monitor you if that is what your surgeon has instructed.

A note of caution: If the medications and methods of pain management you are given cannot control your pain, or if you experience a sudden onset of new pain, contact your plastic surgeon.

96. How can I camouflage the signs that I have had surgery?

Facial procedures

In the first few days following any surgical facial procedure, large-framed sunglasses, a fashionable scarf, or even a hat can be good camouflage. In the following days, there are some very specific cosmetics available to camouflage the bruising or discoloration you may experience. Your plastic surgeon may provide you with camouflage cosmetics, or you may wish to visit the cosmetic counter in a department store or salon. It is sometimes helpful to experiment with camouflage products prior to surgery. But don't use cosmetics on any open wounds postoperatively.

Procedures of the breast

The easiest camouflage for breast procedures is a simple button-down blouse or shirt, or a zip-front sweatshirt. You won't want to be pulling anything over your head in those first few days after surgery. A shirt, even one that is more fitted, will easily conceal a support bra or any swelling. Shop for and set aside these items and a few support bras, in varying styles, prior to your surgery. Cotton bras are generally more comfortable during healing, as is a front closure. Make certain you don't purchase bras or support garments with underwires until you are advised you may wear them. When you are ready to wear a swimsuit, one that is more athletic in design or with a built-in shelf bra will likely be more comfortable, more flattering, and provide more coverage.

Body contouring procedures

With any body contouring procedure, loose-fitting clothing can easily camouflage any swelling. If you have a procedure that significantly reduces the size of your body, shop for some clothing in varying sizes before your procedure. Just make certain that any items you don't wear can be returned.

97. Can I have more than one procedure at a time?

Multiple procedures are commonly performed together, but certain precautions should be taken. Undergoing several extensive procedures at the same time can significantly increase the duration of surgery and anesthesia. Procedures that take longer than six hours increase the risk of infection and pulmonary emboli, and should be performed in a hospital setting or in an accredited facility with overnight care. In addition, large volume liposuction should not be performed with other major, unrelated procedures. This combination can increase your risk for serious, potentially life-threatening complications. Certain surgical combinations work well, others do not. Discuss your alternatives carefully with your plastic surgeon and create a strategic plan to achieve your goals.

98. What procedures are commonly performed together?

Procedures that are generally appropriate to be performed together are those that do not:

- Require multiple positions or draping changes during surgery
- Result in large amounts of blood loss
- Have the potential for contaminating areas that must remain sterile
- Require inordinate amounts of time

Complementary procedures (those that go well together) include:

- Minimally invasive procedures that can often be safely performed with one another or with certain invasive procedures.
- Procedures in the same general anatomic location; for instance, facelift can appropriately be accompanied by brow lift, eyelid surgery, and facial implantation.
- Procedures in different sites (breast and eyelid, for example) where there is no need for repositioning and the procedures are not overly long.
- Other procedure combinations as determined by you and your surgeon.

If you do wish to undergo multiple procedures, fully discuss all of your desires with your plastic surgeon. Then make your decision based on the advantages and disadvantages of having these multiple procedures performed at the same time.

99. Can procedures be repeated?

We know that patients may undergo revisional surgeries for minor problems, such as thickened scars or slight asymmetries. Additionally, the human body continues to age. Therefore, after a period of time, changes will occur in the face and body that may warrant further surgery to achieve more youthful contours. Facial rejuvenation, for instance, will bring you back about 10 years, but 8 to 10 years after surgery, you will see aging that may warrant further surgery. Undergoing another procedure at this time can be very helpful to maintain your more youthful and smooth appearance. It is a good idea for you to know your options for long-range maintenance before you begin treatment.

In 2003, 32% of all plastic surgery patients underwent multiple procedures in one session, according to the American Society of Plastic Surgeons.

100. What if I am not pleased with the outcome of my plastic surgery?

If you are not pleased with your outcome, you first need to discuss this with your plastic surgery provider. Questions to ask yourself and to discuss with your provider include:

• Why am I not pleased?
• Is this my final outcome, or will my results continue to improve?
• What exactly were my expectations for a final outcome, and how have those not been met?

Recovery and Outcomes

- Is my lack of fulfillment with my final result something that I was aware could occur and consented to, or is this something I fully did not expect?
- What can be done to help me achieve what I had hoped would be my outcome?

If you feel you are not getting answers you are comfortable with or wish to seek additional advice, do so. Consult with a like provider and focus on the questions above. But don't expect that provider to tell you something went wrong. A physician will only tell you what can be done to help you meet your goals, if in fact your goals can be met.

The American Society for Aesthetic Plastic Surgery reported in their 2003 procedural statistics a 293% increase in the total number of cosmetic procedures since 1997. An independent study conducted by Synorate and reported by ASAPS in 2003, found that 54% of all Americans approve of cosmetic plastic surgery and 24% would consider it themselves. While this data shows a genuine interest in cosmetic plastic surgery, patient safety and satisfaction can best be achieved in the care of a qualified provider.

The Future, Your Future

What does the future hold for plastic surgery? Much like any field of medicine, the future of plastic surgery holds advances in care, safety, and outcomes. But also, much like any consumer-driven industry, the future of plastic surgery holds advances to meet consumer demands. Today, these demands are focused on natural, long-lasting outcomes with reduced recovery time.

The Future

Plastic surgery techniques, technology, and products are constantly being developed and refined to achieve the most aesthetically-pleasing outcomes possible. At the same time, the goal is to create a natural appearance, where there is balance, or "harmony" among the different components of the face or between the face and body.

With the advent of newer products and technologies, including such things as Botox® and newer injectable soft tissue filler enhancements and cooler lasers, patients are opting for minimally invasive procedures at an earlier age. Additionally, when surgery is necessary to produce a desired outcome, the combination of surgery with the minimally invasive procedures helps to achieve balance and maintain results for longer periods of time.

Minimally invasive rejuvenative procedures are in great demand. At the present time, in the U.S., there are only a few soft-tissue filler substances approved by the Food & Drug Administration, with a few more in the process of approval and many more in off-label use. This is occurring 2 decades after the introduction of bovine collagen to the market. Across Europe and Asia, there are presently over 60 different types of approved fillers on the market, and pharmaceutical companies worldwide are feverishly trying to develop, test, and market better products.

Body contouring techniques and liposuction technology also continue to expand and improve. And breast surgery is ever-changing; the quest for breast implants that are both safe and natural is an on-going international project that seeks to meet the enormous demand for breast enhancement and reconstruction.

Silicone gel breast implants were again submitted to the U.S. FDA for approval in aesthetic breast augmentation in 2003, over a decade after being removed from the market for breast augmentation. The reason for the persistence of the manufacturers and many plastic surgeons is that they, along with many patients, believe that silicone gel-filled implants have a more natural feel and appearance than saline-filled breast implants.

But silicone is not the only breast implant that you may hear about in the future. Manufacturers and plastic surgeons are testing all sorts of new breast implant fillers. At the time this book was released, the same researchers who introduced and tested Trilucent™ breast implants in 1996 had recently patented a breast implant filled with polyethelene glycol (PEG) and saline, and applied to the U.S. FDA to begin using it in clinical trials. It is likely that other combinations of substances are under study, or are currently being developed.

With advances in body surgery and facial technologies, multiple combinations of procedures can be used to create a pleasing total package. But the maintenance of good outcomes depends a great deal upon up-to-date medical and dental care, good skin care and a healthy diet and exercise program.

And, above all else, it is imperative that you learn as much as possible about the qualifications and credentials of your provider and of the facility in which any procedure is to be performed. This is truly an industry of "buyer beware." You cannot "return" a purchase of plastic surgery the way you can return a bad outfit or pair of shoes. For example, consider the number of physicians names, techniques, and surgeons (including unqualified providers) marketing "lunchtime" or minimally invasive facelifts. These procedures are often purported to have equal results to traditional procedures, in less time with minimal risk and fast, pain-free recovery. Although these procedures may provide some improvements, there is still risk and recovery time associated with surgery. And they are known to be less effective and long-lasting than a SMAS facelift. These providers make these claims and market their techniques to appeal to consumer demand. They are allowed to do so despite the fact that the procedures are unproven because these techniques are not reviewed nor approved by the FDA or any other government agency. Furthermore at present, there is no proof that these procedures have met standards for safety or outcomes.

Consumer demand and treatment options will continue to grow. So will the choice of providers. Any licensed physician, even those who have had no surgical training, can market him- or herself as a "plastic" or "cosmetic" surgeon. The government does not intervene here, because these terms are considered to be "generic".

Such actions have drawn attention, however, both by consumers and state regulators, as evidenced by medical truth in advertising legislation, as discussed in Part 2 of this book. It is of utmost importance that you choose qualified and appropriate providers who are board-certified by appropriate American Board of Medical Specialties boards.

Your Future

If you choose to have plastic surgery now or in the future, you will hopefully use this book as a tool to help you identify your desire, choose a qualified provider, and with the guidance of that provider, make a decision that is right for you. Plastic surgery is your choice; it is your decision. Make it an educated choice and a confident decision, for today and for your future. Don't make your choice of treatment or provider based on marketing appeals. Choose a provider for any surgical or minimally-invasive procedure based on training credentials, and experience in both traditional methods and minimally invasive procedures.

While we cannot state in numbers how plastic surgery affects the lives of individual patients, we can state with great confidence that plastic surgery is most often immensely satisfying for good candidates, with realistic expectations, in the care of qualified providers. How do we know this? Look at the growing number of plastic surgery procedures performed each year, and the growing number of plastic surgery patients. Logic will tell you these people are fulfilled. Growing numbers of educated, informed, and confident individuals do not undergo elective medical procedures—plastic surgery, and more importantly, procedures that are accompanied in every case by the potential for discomfort and risk—unless the greater odds are, that plastic surgery is likely to fulfill their goals.

If you are considering plastic surgery, approach your interest with realistic goals, with careful consideration, and with confidence in yourself. Plastic surgery alone cannot change who you are, or change your life. It can, however, enhance your appearance and your confidence. Only you can change your life.

Index

Index

Jasper County Public Library System

Overdue notices are a courtesy of
the library system.
Failure to receive an overdue notice
does not absolve the borrower of the
obligation to return materials on time.

DEMCO